Surgical Atlas of
Gynecologic
Oncology

Surgical Atlas of Gynecologic Oncology

Donald G. Gallup, M.D.

Professor and Director
Section of Gynecologic Oncology
Department of Obstetrics and Gynecology
Medical College of Georgia
Augusta, Georgia

O. Eduardo Talledo, M.D.

Director, Gynecologic Oncology
Savannah Memorial Medical Center
Savannah, Georgia

Illustrations by

Elizabeth Boardman Berry

W.B. SAUNDERS COMPANY
A Division of Harcourt Brace & Company
Philadelphia   London   Toronto   Montreal   Sydney   Tokyo

W.B. SAUNDERS COMPANY
A Division of
Harcourt Brace & Company

The Curtis Center
Independence Square West
Philadelphia, Pennsylvania 19106

Library of Congress Cataloging-in-Publication Data

Surgical atlas of gynecologic oncology /
[edited by] Donald G. Gallup, O. Eduardo Talledo.—1st ed.

p. cm.

ISBN 0–7216–3980–1

1. Generative organs, Female—Cancer—Surgery—
   Atlases.   I. Gallup, Donald G.   II. Talledo,
   O. Eduardo.   [DNLM: 1. Genital Neoplasms,
   Female—surgery—atlases.   WP 17 S961 1994]

RG104.6. S926 1994   616.99′465059—dc20

DNLM/DLC   93–32871

SURGICAL ATLAS OF GYNECOLOGIC ONCOLOGY   ISBN 0–7216–3980–1

Last digit is the print number: 9   8   7   6   5   4   3   2   1

Contributors

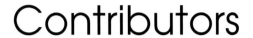

Donald G. Gallup, M.D.
  Professor and Director, Section of Gynecologic Oncology, Department of
  Obstetrics and Gynecology, Medical College of Georgia, Augusta, Georgia

Deborah L. Coleman Gallup, M.D.
  Assistant Professor, Department of Obstetrics and Gynecology, Medical College
  of Georgia, Augusta, Georgia

Laurel A. King, M.D.
  Assistant Professor, Gynecologic Oncology, Medical College of Georgia,
  Augusta, Georgia

Mark J. Messing, M.D.
  Associate Professor, Section of Gynecologic Oncology, Department of
  Obstetrics and Gynecology, Medical College of Georgia, Augusta, Georgia

Thomas E. Nolan, M.D.
  Associate Professor, Departments of Obstetrics and Gynecology and Internal
  Medicine, Louisiana State University School of Medicine, New Orleans,
  Louisiana

O. Eduardo Talledo, M.D.
  Director, Gynecologic Oncology, Savannah Memorial Medical Center,
  Savannah, Georgia

Preface

Over the past several decades, formal fellowship programs and eventual subspecialization in gynecologic oncology have led to a modern era of pelvic surgery for cancer of the female genital tract. Technological advances have led to better preoperative and postoperative care and have provided a variety of surgical instruments and sutures that have contributed to decreased operative time and morbidity. Large retrospective studies and prospective studies from such organizations as the Gynecologic Oncology Group have evaluated some of the more radical procedures performed in the past. As a result, certain gynecologic malignancies can be safely managed with less disfiguring operative procedures. In addition, reconstructive techniques have been developed that have improved the quality of life and thus acceptance for women undergoing ultraradical procedures.

Our purpose in writing this *Surgical Atlas of Gynecologic Oncology* is to record the majority of procedures used by gynecologic oncologists in managing female genital tract malignancies. We have attempted to blend the "old" and the "new" by emphasizing less radical surgery when deemed appropriate. Although some of the complications of gynecologic malignancies, such as vesicovaginal and rectovaginal fistulas, have been addressed, this atlas does not include routine gynecologic procedures, nor is it intended to include all bowel or urinary tract operations.

The authors have spent countless hours at the operating table with each other in developing some of these techniques. However, the procedures described herein are a modification of techniques taught to all of us by masters from institutions throughout the country, such as the University of Michigan, University of Minnesota, M.D. Anderson Hospital in Houston, and Memorial Sloan-Kettering Cancer Center. This atlas as conceived is an accumulation of knowledge we have gained from our many mentors over the years. We are thus indebted to the teaching of the master surgeons at these and other institutions: William E. Lucas, George W. Morley, Ernst Navatril, Joe V. Meigs, Alexander Brunschwig, and George F. McInnes. The atlas represents a summation of the many talents of those who have gone before us.

We would like to express our gratitude to our medical illustrators, headed by Elizabeth Boardman-Berry and including Charles Boyter, Karen Waldo, Milton Burroughs, and David Mascaro. Their skillful art translated our surgical techniques into beautiful, comprehensible drawings. We recognize our secretaries, Debbie Johnson, Anne Todd, and Nora McClendon, for preparation of the manuscript.

Our final thanks are to our publisher, the W. B. Saunders Company, and to the medical editor of this atlas, Avé McCracken, whose encouragement and gentle prodding have led to the fruition of this teaching aid.

DONALD G. GALLUP, M.D.
O. EDUARDO TALLEDO, M.D.

Contents

1

Perioperative Management of the Surgical Patient and
Central Line Placement Techniques   1

Thomas E. Nolan, M.D.

2

Alternate Surgical Procedures for Early Vulvar Carcinoma   25

3

Radical Vulvectomy and Groin Dissection   33

4

Abdominal Incisions and Closures   43

5

Extraperitoneal Pelvic Lymph Node Dissection with
Modified Radical Hysterectomy   53

6

Radical Hysterectomy with Pelvic Lymph Node Dissection   65

7

Surgery for Advanced Ovarian Cancer   87

Mark J. Messing, M.D.

8

Extraperitoneal Approaches to Para-aortic Nodes   107

9

Transperitoneal Approach to the Para-aortic
Lymph Nodes   125

Mark J. Messing, M.D.

10

Total Pelvic Exenteration   139

11

Anterior and Posterior Pelvic Exenteration   163

Mark J. Messing, M.D.

12

The Continent Urinary Reservoir   183

Laurel A. King, M.D.

13

Repair of Vesicovaginal Fistulas and Operative Injuries
to the Distal Ureter   195

14

Rectovaginal Fistula   207

15

The Use of Locally Mobilized Skin (Z-Plasty and
Rhomboid Flaps) for Large Defects   223

Deborah L. Coleman Gallup, M.D.

16

Gracilis Myocutaneous Flap   231

17

The Tensor Fascia Lata Flap   239

Laurel A. King, M.D.

18

Alternate Reconstructive Techniques for Repair of
Large Vulvar and Vaginal Defects   249

Laurel A. King, M.D.

Index   263

1

Perioperative Management of the Surgical Patient and Central Line Placement Techniques

Thomas E. Nolan, M.D.

The difference between the good surgeon and the great surgeon is the attention to detail in the perioperative period.

The outcome of any surgical case begins with a well-conceived preoperative plan that accounts for both the medical aspects of the patient and the surgical approach. Additionally, technically superb surgery can quickly be reversed by a poorly managed postoperative course. The surgical patient who presents with chronic disease requires a special preoperative work-up to better quantitate the impact surgery will have on major organ systems and nutrition. The work-up should focus on the ability of the patient to withstand physiologic stress. In the postoperative period, the patient with underlying systemic diseases may become overwhelmed by immobilization, anesthetics, and narcotics. A well thought out postoperative management plan may help decrease morbidity. Additionally, an extensive review of systems may uncover previously undiagnosed medical diseases that may contribute to intraoperative and postoperative morbidity.

HISTORY AND PHYSICAL EXAMINATION

Cardiovascular Disease

Cardiovascular disease may contribute significantly to perioperative morbidity and mortality. With aging, various systemic diseases are more prevalent and affect cardiac reserve. Three major cardiac disease states should be considered: (1) coronary artery disease with special emphasis on perioperative myocardial infarction; (2) valvular heart disease, especially in patients who have stenotic lesions and do not tolerate excessive fluid volumes; and (3) hypertension, which may predispose to several problems, including myocardial infarction and stroke.

Coronary artery disease becomes more prevalent with aging. Patients who suffer from chronic hypertension, or who have a decrease in high-density lipoprotein (HDL) cholesterol, with a sedentary lifestyle and obesity, may be a prime set-up for myocardial infarction. A family history of early myocardial infarctions (younger than 55 years old) may signal the presence of a hyperlipidemia. Any postmenopausal patient with a chest pain history, regardless of how atypical, deserves further evaluation. The diabetic patient is at high risk for "silent" myocardial ischemia owing to commonly associated neuropathy. Poor diabetic control is associated with unfavorable lipid status and predisposes to atherosclerosis. Adequate assessment of cardiovascular reserves in high-risk patients is mandatory.

Valvular heart disease is associated with many potential perioperative complications. Patients with stenotic lesions may handle increased fluid volumes poorly. The two most common lesions seen are mitral stenosis, usually secondary to rheumatic heart disease, and aortic stenosis (or sclerosis due to calcifications secondary to atherosclerosis), noted frequently in the elderly patient. A history of dyspnea on exertion or orthopnea should lead to an evaluation for valvular heart disease. A relatively common condition in women is mitral valve prolapse, which may require antibiotic prophylaxis perioperatively. The echocardiogram has become an excellent noninvasive tool to evaluate valvular heart disease.

Hypertension is especially prevalent in the female patient older than 50 years of age. To be significant as a predictor of perioperative morbidity, a level of 170/110 mmHg must be reached. Side effects of various medications may have important ramifications in the operative time period. Diuretics, especially the loop diuretics, may decrease intravascular volume and contribute to fluid management problems. Sudden withdrawal of beta blockers has precipitated angina in patients with underlying coronary artery disease. Prior to surgery, long-acting preparations of beta blockers may be substituted, or nitroglycerin paste or patches may be used until oral intake is begun. The patient receiving calcium channel blockers may require a change in medication to long-acting agents during the perioperative period owing to a lack of parenteral preparations. Theoretical concerns were initially raised regarding the use of angiotensin converting enzyme (ACE) inhibitors and associated hypovolemia, which could be easily reversed by volume expansion. In actual practice, hypotension has not developed, and currently ACE inhibitors are continued until surgery. Additionally, an intravenous ACE inhibitor preparation (enalaprilat) is now available for use in the postoperative course. Patients requiring smooth muscle relaxants, such as hydralazine and minoxidil, may require nitroglycerin or nitroprusside during induction and when awaking from anesthesia.

The physical examination for cardiovascular disease should be directed toward evidence of poor left ventricular performance. Patients who have suffered multiple myocardial infarctions, who have cardiomyopathies, who have valvular heart disease, or who have a history of congestive heart failure need a directed physical examination for evidence of cardiac failure. This includes the presence of neck vein distention at 30 degrees elevation, the presence of rales, and the presence of S_3 and S_4 gallops suggestive of left ventricular failure. The patient who has physical signs suggestive of cardiac failure or who gives a history of prior pulmonary edema or congestive heart failure should be considered for central vein access with or without a pulmonary artery catheter to better assess fluid management.

Blood pressure assessment and control should be documented. The patient with new-onset hypertension should be treated for at least 3 weeks prior to surgery to allow for compensatory mechanisms, such as the baroreceptors, to compensate. Patients on multiple antihypertensive medications should be evaluated to simplify their regimens, if possible. Assessment of volume status by performing a "tilt test" should be performed for patients on loop diuretics.

Some elderly patients are limited by disease in the amount of exercise they can perform. These patients should be tested for cardiac reserve. A poor prognosticator for surgery is the inability of a patient to increase heart rate to greater than 99 beats per minute with exercise. If the patient lacks the ability to increase the heart rate, additional testing of cardiovascular reserve and the presence of coronary artery disease should be considered.

Pulmonary Diseases

Pulmonary problems and diseases are common in the perioperative period. Risk factors for postoperative pulmonary complications are found in Table 1–1. Chronic obstructive pulmonary disease (COPD), bronchospastic disease, and cigarette-induced bronchitis are common conditions that may contribute to postoperative problems. Pulmonary function tests (PFTs) should be ordered in patients with a history of dyspnea on exertion or a history of any chronic pulmonary disease. The routine performance of

Table 1–1. RISK FACTORS FOR POSTOPERATIVE PULMONARY COMPLICATIONS

- Age >70 years
- Cigarette smoking (especially over 40 pack-years)
- Pre-existing pulmonary disease
- Excessive sputum production
- Obesity > 120% of expected weight
- Location of surgical procedure (upper abdomen > lower abdomen > vaginal incision)
- Neuromuscular disease (multiple sclerosis and myasthenia gravis)
- P_{CO_2} > 45 torr, P_{O_2} < 70 torr on arterial blood gas
- Spirometric parameters
  FVC < 50% after adjusting for age and sex
  FEV_1/FVC of 65–75% = mildly increased risk
  FEV_1/FVC of 50–65% = moderately increased risk
  FEV_1/FVC of < 50% = markedly increased risk

Abbreviations: FVC = forced vital capacity; FEV_1 = forced expiratory volume at 1 second.

PFTs in patients 70 years of age or older is no longer recommended. A history of cigarette use may be important in guiding the need for preoperative pulmonary function testing. Those patients who have greater than a 40 pack-year history of smoking (pack-years = number of packs consumed per day multiplied by number of years) deserve pulmonary function testing. Arterial blood gases demonstrating a P_{CO_2} greater than 45 mmHg are significantly correlated with postoperative morbidity and mechanical ventilation.

Bronchospastic disease (asthma) sufferers require maintenance therapy during the perioperative period. The routine use of theophyllines has decreased in the last decade and has been replaced by beta-2 aerosols such as albuterol and metaproterenol. These can be given up to the time of surgery and can be administered in the anesthetic circuit during surgery. Patients who have used "chronic" steroids within the past year require perioperative steroids.

Heavy cigarette use is associated with many postoperative pulmonary problems. The chronic inflammatory effects of smoke on the trachea result in an excessive number of goblet cells, which leads to increased secretions. Anesthetic gases and endotracheal tubes decrease ciliary motion in the trachea and therefore impair the ability of secretions to be expelled. These changes contribute to atelectasis and pneumonia. These high-risk patients should be seen by a respiratory therapist prior to surgery.

The pulmonary physical examination should be directed at assessing the impact of cigarette smoking, COPD, and bronchospasm. The cigarette smoker with auscultatory findings of wheezing or rhonchi with a cough is at risk for pulmonary complications. Patients with long-standing bronchospasm and accompanying wheezing should be considered for systemic steroids for stabilization prior to surgery. Patients with well-advanced cases of COPD have an increase in the anterior-posterior thoracic diameter and neck accessory muscle usage. Distant breath sounds, wheezing, and rales are common findings in advanced disease.

Gastrointestinal Diseases

Diseases of the liver may be difficult to diagnose. Patients may be social "alcoholics" who drink excessive quantities of alcohol on a chronic basis and do not consider themselves to be alcoholics. An adequate history of alcohol use should be obtained. Biliary colic and gallbladder diseases are common in postoperative patients. A history of right upper quadrant or mid-epigastric pain should be sought prior to any surgical procedure.

Table 1–2. AUTOSOMAL DOMINANT AND FAMILIAL GASTROINTESTINAL SYNDROMES

Syndrome	Distribution	Malignant Potential
Gardner's syndrome	Large and small intestine	Common
Familial colonic polyposis	Large intestine	Common
Turcot's syndrome	Large intestine	Common
Non-polyposis syndrome	Large intestine	Common
Juvenile polyposis	Stomach, large and small intestine	Rare
Peutz-Jeghers syndrome	Stomach, large and small intestine	Rare
Cancer family syndrome	Large intestine, ovary, endometrium	Common
Ulcerative colitis	Large intestine	Common

A strong family history of colon carcinoma should be explored with preoperative studies. Multiple colon carcinoma syndromes that are associated with systemic diseases or are genetically transmitted have been described (Table 1–2). Patients who present with a pelvic mass and a strong family history of colonic carcinoma should undergo further work-up with an air-contrast barium enema, flexible sigmoidoscopy, or colonoscopy as indicated.

Physical examination of the gastrointestinal tract includes palpation and percussion for identification of hepatosplenomegaly associated with alcoholism or chronic active hepatitis. A rectal examination should be performed with the pelvic examination to evaluate any possible masses. Patients 50 years of age or older should have their stool evaluated for occult blood.

Endocrinology

Thyroid diseases, especially hyperthyroidism, can be unmasked during surgery. A higher prevalence of thyroid disease is seen in women who have first-degree relatives with thyroid problems. Many patients have been diagnosed as hypothyroid and unexpectedly have had their thyroid medication stopped. Such patients require reassessment of their thyroid status prior to surgery. Hypothyroid patients should receive lifetime thyroid replacement. The diabetic patient should be evaluated with special attention given to associated conditions including atherosclerosis, coronary artery disease, chronic renal insufficiency, and hypertension. Any associated disease should be under adequate medical control.

The most common etiology of hypoadrenalism is exogenous steroid use. A careful history of usage of various steroid preparations should be taken preoperatively. Any patient who receives more than 1 week of 7.5 mg daily of prednisone in the previous year will require steroid replacement during the preoperative and postoperative periods.

Thyroid size should be evaluated during the initial physical examination. The presence of exophthalmos with tachycardia, tremor, sleep disorders, and unexplained loss of hair suggests the possibility of Graves' disease. Diabetic patients should be examined for evidence of vascular insufficiency. Surgery should usually be postponed if evidence of chronic foot infections is present.

Renal Insufficiency

The patient who has long-standing hypertension and the elderly patient may have varying degrees of renal insufficiency. The aging patient, at age 65, may have a decrease in creatinine clearance to 75 ml per hour. Patients who give a history of unexpected edema or the inability to tolerate high salt loads should be evaluated for renal problems, as should patients who have received potentially renal toxic drugs.

Obesity

Obesity is defined as 120 per cent of ideal body weight and is associated with multiple cardiopulmonary changes that may have an impact on postoperative management. Ventilation/perfusion abnormalities are related to mechanical problems of chest wall movement. Additionally, these patients have a higher incidence of hypertension, diabetes, and atherosclerosis resulting in coronary artery disease. Preventive methods to avoid deep vein thrombosis and pulmonary embolism should be instituted.

LABORATORY TESTING

The effectiveness of routine laboratory testing has been questioned in the last decade. A complete blood count (CBC) is important to diagnose anemia and plan fluid replacement perioperatively. In the era of acquired immunodeficiency syndrome (AIDS), preoperative work-up and therapy of anemia have achieved a greater significance. The use of routine coagulation tests (prothrombin time [PT], partial thromboplastin time [PTT]) should be discouraged, except in those patients with a known coagulation abnormality or those receiving anticoagulant therapy. The most common reason for a prolonged coagulation test is human variation. If a bleeding diathesis is considered, the bleeding time is a superior test. Despite testing limitations, patients with the most common bleeding diathesis (von Willebrand's disease) will have an abnormal bleeding time.

Examination of serum electrolytes should be individualized to patients who have certain diseases (such as diabetes, hypertension, or known renal disease) or who are taking medications that will have an impact (such as diuretics). Patients with fistulas, known gastrointestinal symptoms, or prior surgeries should be evaluated for electrolyte abnormalities. A urinalysis should be performed to rule out subacute urinary tract infections.

A routine preoperative chest x-ray and electrocardiogram (ECG) should be performed in patients older than 45 years or when warranted by medical condition. In patients with a chest pain history, a more thorough assessment of cardiac function is performed. Owing to the excessive number of false-positive exercise stress tests in women patients, most cardiologists will opt for thallium scanning. It is noninvasive, sensitive, and specific for perfusion abnormalities; however, its major limitation is expense. Coronary angiography, despite its invasive nature and complications (though rare), remains the "gold standard" for evaluation of coronary artery and valvular disease.

Pulmonary function testing is indicated in the cigarette smoker with a greater than 40 pack-year history of use, in the patient with COPD, in the obese patient, in the patient with excessive sputum production, and in the patient with systemic disease, such as one of the connective tissue syndromes. The elderly patient with kyphosis from osteoporosis may have elements of both restrictive and obstructive disease. Routine use of PFTs in patients older than 70 should be discouraged unless directed by the history and physical examination. Additionally, arterial blood gases may be helpful in some patients. A Pco_2 of greater than 45 mmHg is strongly suggestive of significant COPD requiring postoperative mechanical ventilation. The necessity of a surgical procedure may be reevaluated in patients with compromised pulmonary reserves, particularly when other options such as radiotherapy or chemotherapy may be efficacious.

Imaging

The use of imaging in obstetrics and gynecology is becoming more common. In addition to the use of chest x-rays, intravenous pyelography, and occasionally barium enemas in cervical cancer work-ups,

computed tomographic scanning (CT scan) and vaginal probe ultrasonography can be used to assess adnexal masses. Lymphangiography is probably the most sensitive radiographic method to assess lymph node status in patients with known female genital tract malignancies. Serum testing for tumor markers (CA-125, etc.) combined with imaging may help in deciding when to refer the patient to a gynecologic oncologist. Preoperative markers are often helpful in management of patients with ovarian malignancies. Patients who have guaiac-positive stools or suspicious lower pelvic masses with possible colonic involvement should undergo air-contrast barium enema with flexible sigmoidoscopy or colonoscopy.

Not all masses require imaging. This is particularly true of patients with midline masses, clinically consistent with leiomyomata. The patient with an obvious midline mass consistent with leiomyomata uteri does not need imaging. Intravenous pyelography (IVP) should be considered in patients with a history of an adnexal mass, endometriosis, or severe pelvic inflammatory disease. The routine use of IVP should be discouraged because of minimal benefit, the known disadvantages of their cost, and risk of death caused by allergies to the dye used in IVP.

Invasive Monitoring

The establishment of intensive care units has contributed to the popularity of invasive monitoring. Catheterization of peripheral arteries ("a-lines") is done for frequent assessment of oxygenation and laboratory measurements. Common indications for a-line placement include the necessity of extensive surgery, expected intensive care unit care in compromised patients, and sometimes poor vascular access, especially in the elderly patient.

In the past 15 years, the use of pulmonary artery catheters (PAC) has become common in the United States. The indications for pulmonary artery catheters should be considered during the preoperative evaluation. Central venous access should be performed prior to surgery if pulmonary artery catheter use is indicated or considered. The routine placement of pulmonary artery catheters should be discouraged. Table 1–3 reviews the indications for use of pulmonary artery catheters.

General Principles in Central Venous Access

Large central veins are used for access when peripheral veins are no longer available or when long-term therapy is necessary. The surgical area should

Table 1–3. INDICATIONS FOR PULMONARY ARTERY CATHETERIZATION IN OBSTETRICS AND GYNECOLOGY

I. Cardiac Disease/Dysfunction
  • History of pulmonary edema, congestive heart failure, or compromised left ventricular function (ejection fraction < 40%)
  • Severe valvular heart disease (usually stenotic or atretic lesions)
  • Cardiomyopathy with ejection fraction < 40%
II. Pulmonary Disease/Dysfunction
  • Management of fluids with positive end expiratory pressure > 15 mmHg in adult respiratory distress syndrome
  • Progressive pulmonary edema/hypoxemia
III. Renal Dysfunction
  • Persistent oliguria/renal failure despite volume challenge and afterload reduction (e.g., severe pre-eclampsia)
IV. Sequelae of Systemic Infection
  • Septic shock, regardless of etiology, refractory to standard volume and pressor therapies

be prepped and draped, using sterile technique. Most central lines are placed for a minimum of 3 to 7 days, making asepsis mandatory. Adequate anesthesia is a prerequisite owing to the anatomic location. The Seldinger technique of inserting a large-bore catheter over a previously placed guide wire is commonly used. Once the procedure is completed, a chest radiograph is obtained to inspect catheter position and to observe any complications (pneumothorax, etc.)

Central Access of the Internal Jugular Vein Using the Anterior Triangle Approach

Central line placement is usually done in one of two locations. Patients who are undergoing short-term intensive care can be adequately managed with insertion via the internal jugular vein. The most significant complication from this approach is a carotid artery catheterization, but the chance of this complication can be minimized by retracting the carotid artery medially during insertion. Patients requiring long-term therapy should be managed by the subclavian approach, which is anatomically more stable and comfortable to the patient than use of the internal jugular vein but has the additional complications of hemo- and pneumothorax. The techniques for placement of these two central venous access lines are noted in Figures 1–1 through 1–18.

THERAPIES FOR THE PERIOPERATIVE PATIENT

Prophylactic Antibiotics

The use of prophylactic antibiotics in vaginal surgery is well established. Their efficacy in simple transabdominal hysterectomy has not been widely accepted. However, for prolonged procedures, such as radical hysterectomy, several studies suggest that they can be beneficial. The first-generation cephalosporins are sufficient for routine prophylaxis and work by lowering the number of organisms in operative sites. These give adequate coverage of the common pathogens in gynecologic surgery. Prophylactic antibiotics should be given shortly (approximately 1 hour) prior to the initiation of surgery. Many surgeons still continue to use two doses postoperatively, the first 2 hours after surgery and a second dose 8 hours later.

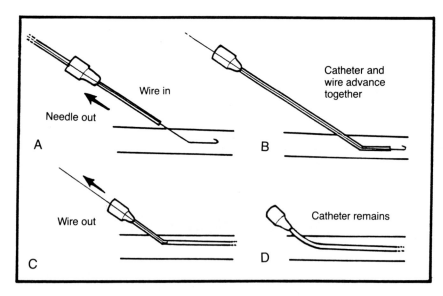

Figure 1–1. The Seldinger technique is the most common method used to catheterize both arterial vessels and for central venous access. A small seeker needle identifies the artery or vein to be catheterized, followed by a guide wire, and finally the permanent catheter is placed over the wire.

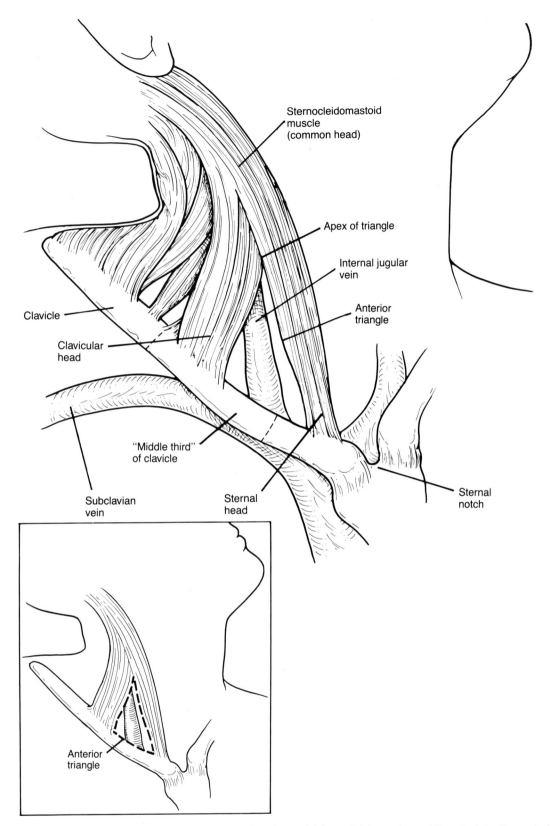

Sternocleidomastoid muscle (common head)

Apex of triangle

Internal jugular vein

Anterior triangle

Clavicle

Clavicular head

"Middle third" of clavicle

Sternal notch

Subclavian vein

Sternal head

Anterior triangle

Figure 1–2. The anterior triangle of the neck is created by the sternocleidomastoid muscle and the clavicle. The anterior border consists of the sternal head of the sternocleidomastoid muscle; the posterior border consists of the clavicular head of the sternocleidomastoid muscle; and the inferior border is created by the clavicle. The meeting of sternal and clavicular heads is commonly referred to as either the apex or the "crotch" of the triangle. The sternal notch is identified, and the clavicle is divided into thirds. The patient's head should be positioned in the direction opposite that of the attempted catheterization. If the neck muscles are not easily seen, a towel should be placed between the scapula.

The internal jugular vein is lateral to the carotid artery. Palpation of the carotid artery should be performed prior to any invasive maneuvers. Many operators find that retracting the carotid medially is beneficial (and reassuring) while attempting catheterization.

7

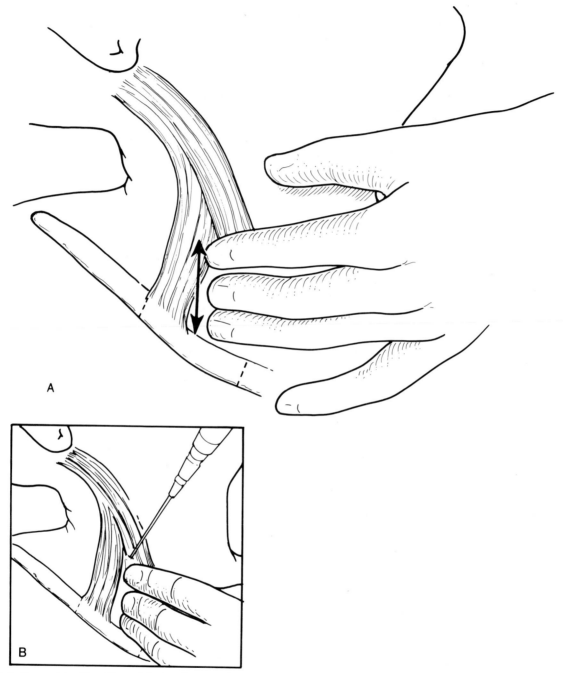

Figure 1–3. The point of insertion of the seeker needle is approximately three finger's breadths superior to the clavicle in the woman patient. In the thin patient, the junction of the two bellies of the sternocleidomastoid muscle is easily recognized; however, in the obese patient it may be found only by palpation.

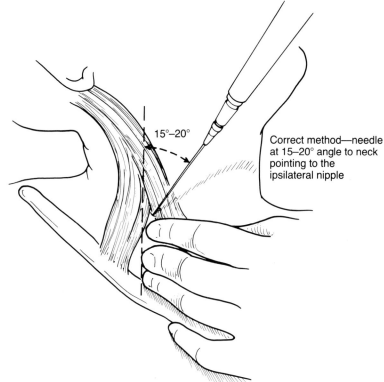

15°–20°

Correct method—needle at 15–20° angle to neck pointing to the ipsilateral nipple

Figure 1–4. The seeker needle is positioned above the third finger for entry into the internal jugular vein. The carotid artery is palpated and retracted medially. The needle is ''aimed'' in the direction of the ipsilateral nipple. Notice the angle of needle in relationship to the skin and anterior triangle of the neck. The proper angle of insertion of the seeker needle should be 15 to 20° from the imaginary midline. Several common mistakes are often made while learning this technique. First, the angle of the needle is too medial, and inadvertent carotid catheterization takes place. Second, the angle to the skin when advancing the seeker needle is not proper, and the needle ''slides'' down the fascia. Pneumothorax may result, most commonly when the apex of the lung is hyperinflated from COPD.

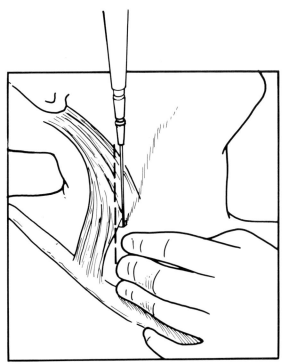

Incorrect method— needle parallel to neck

Figure 1–5. The seeker needle is too medial, and inadvertent carotid catheterization may occur. Additionally, the needle hub is lowered to a less acute angle to the skin. This may result in a pneumothorax, especially in the patient with COPD with a hyperinflated apex of the lung. Once the seeker needle catheterizes the internal jugular, it should be advanced 1 to 2 mm, and the hub of the syringe and the needle are moved to a position parallel to the neck to allow for an easy insertion of the guide wire. Aspiration of blood should be performed a second time and the blood should be free flowing.

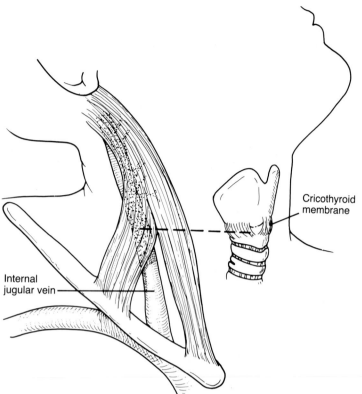

Cricothyroid
membrane

Internal
jugular vein

Figure 1-6. Obese patients present special difficulties owing to a loss of visible landmarks. The cricothyroid fascia should be identified in the midline of the neck superior to the thyroid.

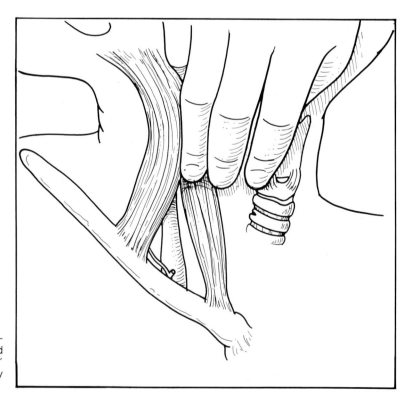

Figure 1-7. Lateral to the cricothyroid, three fingers are placed perpendicular to the cricothyroid fascia. This is approximately where the ``crotch'' or apex of the anterior triangle is anatomically located.

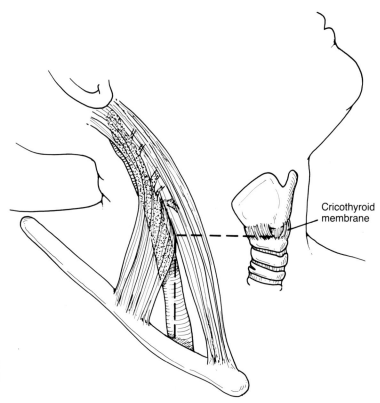

Cricothyroid
membrane

Figure 1–8. In most patients, an imaginary point can be traced by using landmarks from the cricothyroid membrane and the clavicle.

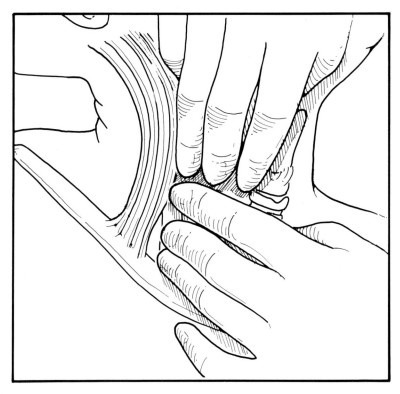

Figure 1–9. By combining this point with three finger's breadths superior to the clavicle, the region of the anterior triangle is identified. The seeker needle should be placed as described earlier.

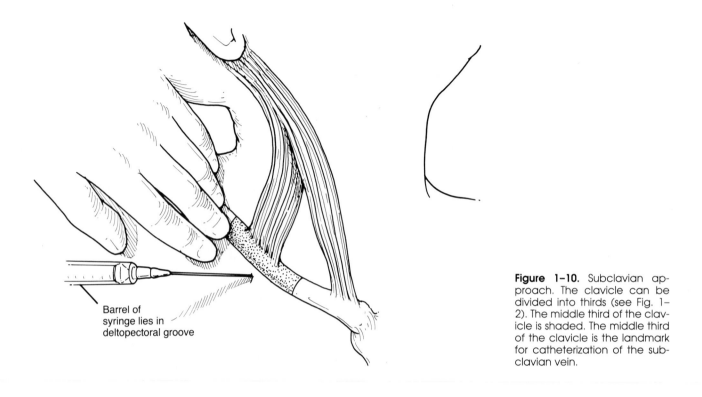

Barrel of
syringe lies in
deltopectoral groove

Figure 1-10. Subclavian approach. The clavicle can be divided into thirds (see Fig. 1-2). The middle third of the clavicle is shaded. The middle third of the clavicle is the landmark for catheterization of the subclavian vein.

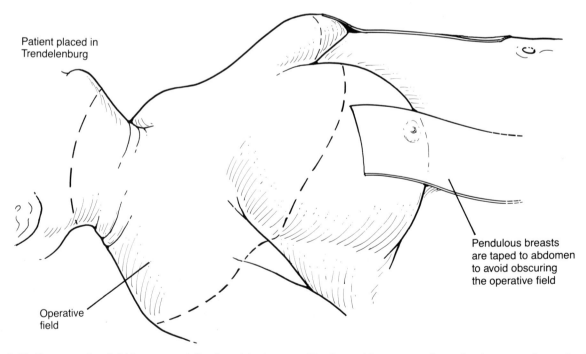

Patient placed in
Trendelenburg

Pendulous breasts
are taped to abdomen
to avoid obscuring
the operative field

Operative
field

Figure 1-11. The operative field is prepared. The Trendelenburg position is used to engorge the veins; however, the patient with pendulous breasts may have distorted anatomy. Taping the breasts inferiorly will allow for an unobscured operative field.

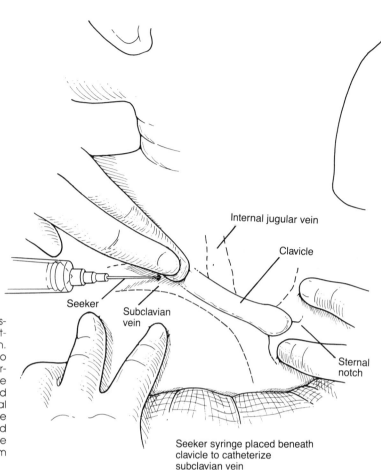

Internal jugular vein

Clavicle

Seeker

Subclavian vein

Sternal notch

Seeker syringe placed beneath clavicle to catheterize subclavian vein

Figure 1–12. The periosteum should be well anesthetized with 1 to 2 per cent xylocaine prior to attempting catheterization of the subclavian vein. The skin is entered approximately 2 cm caudad to the clavicle. The needle and syringe should be parallel to the skin with the barrel of the syringe in the deltoid-pectoral groove. The seeker needle should be aimed toward the manubrium of the sternal notch. Once the skin has been entered, the needle is advanced to the periosteum. Pressure is applied to the skin above the needle while advancing the needle, which should prevent the needle tip from puncturing the lung beneath the clavicle.

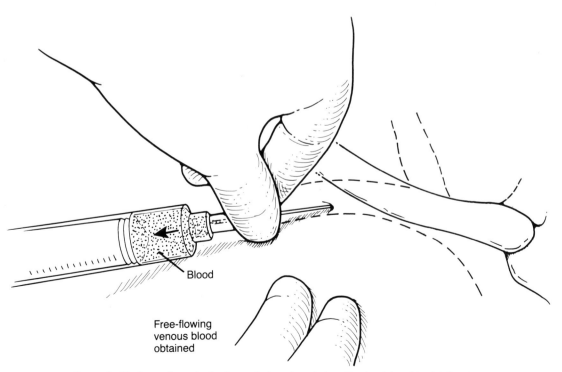

Blood

Free-flowing venous blood obtained

Figure 1–13. Once the subclavian vein is entered, free-flowing blood is obtained.

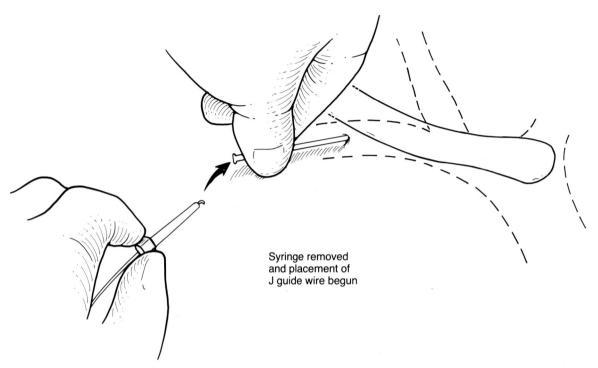

Syringe removed
and placement of
J guide wire begun

Figure 1–14. After the vein is catheterized, a J guide wire is placed with the loop facing inferiorly and threaded to the superior vena cava.

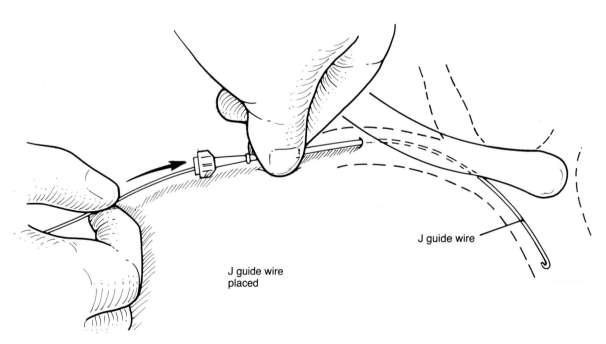

J guide wire
placed

J guide wire

Figure 1–15. The J guide wire is in place in the superior vena cava. Note that the J portion of wire is positioned to "hook" into the vena cava from the subclavian vein.

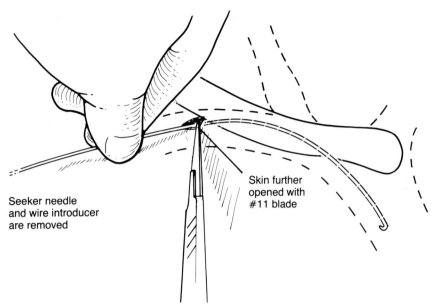

Seeker needle
and wire introducer
are removed

Skin further
opened with
#11 blade

Figure 1-16. An incision has been made for the placement of the vein dilator and introducer. The needle and syringe have been previously removed.

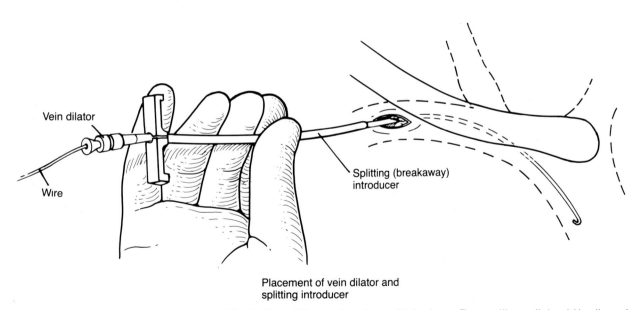

Vein dilator

Wire

Splitting (breakaway)
introducer

Placement of vein dilator and
splitting introducer

Figure 1-17. The vein dilator should be placed inside the splitting (or breakaway) introducer. The resulting unit should be threaded over the guide wire and introduced through the previously made incision. The end of the guide wire should **never be released while the introducer is threaded!!**

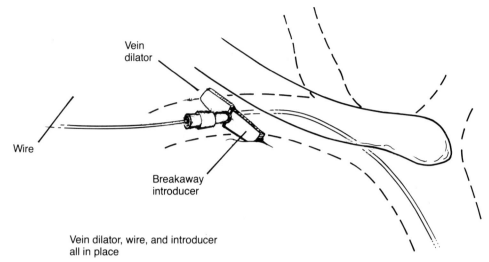

Vein
dilator

Wire

Breakaway
introducer

Vein dilator, wire, and introducer
all in place

Figure 1-18. The introducer, vein dilator, and guide wire are in place. The vein dilator and guide wire are removed, leaving only the breakaway introducer. A catheter can then be inserted as shown in Figure 1-19.

Cardiovascular

Cardiac medications used in the perioperative period should be discussed with the cardiologist and anesthesiologist prior to surgery. Multiple medications with long half-lives have been introduced. If at all possible, the patient should be given antihypertensives and anti-anginal medications prior to surgery with a sip of water. Many patients do not require the degree of hypertensive control in the first 24 to 48 hours postoperatively as they did preoperatively. Common complications in patients with cardiac disease are congestive heart failure and myocardial infarction. Congestive heart failure occurs in the first 48 hours postoperatively and is due to fluid overload intraoperatively or during the mobilization of third-space fluid. Myocardial infarction occurs most commonly on the sixth postoperative day.

The most recent guidelines for antibiotic prophylaxis from the American Heart Association are found in Tables 1-4 and 1-5.

Antihypertensive medications given in the perioperative period should be individualized. Patients on diuretics do not usually require these medications in the first 48 hours following surgery. After 48 hours, diuresis of intraoperative fluid loads and third-space fluids begins to mobilize. Patients with a compromised left ventricle are susceptible to pulmonary edema during this phase, and diuretics should be reinstituted (e.g., intravenous furosemide). Abrupt withdrawal of beta blockers may precipitate angina in patients with coronary insufficiency, and long-acting preparations (Inderal LA, etc.) should begin prior to surgery or nitroglycerin patches should be substituted. Clonidine withdrawal has been associated with severe rebound hypertension. Long-acting clonidine patches can be substituted for oral preparations but should be initiated approximately 48 hours prior to surgery. There are many long-acting oral calcium channel blockers (diltiazem slow release, nifedipine extended release) that can be used in patients who require these for both angina and antihypertension control. Additionally, the new ACE inhibitors now have an IV preparation (enalaprilat) that can be given every 6 hours. Intravenous nitroprusside or nitroglycerin can be substituted for the smooth muscle relaxants (prazosin) acutely.

Table 1-4. RECOMMENDATIONS ON PROPHYLAXIS FOR CARDIAC CONDITIONS

Prophylaxis Recommended
- Prosthetic cardiac valves, including biosynthetic and homograft valves
- Previous bacterial endocarditis, despite absence of heart disease
- Most congenital malformations
- Rheumatic and acquired valvular dysfunction despite repair
- Hypertrophic cardiomyopathy
- Mitral valve prolapse with regurgitation

Prophylaxis Not Recommended
- Isolated secundum atrial septal defect
- Surgical repair without residual beyond 6 months of secundum atrial or ventricular septal defect, or patent ductus arteriosus
- Previous coronary artery bypass surgery
- Mitral valve prolapse without regurgitation
- Innocent or physiologic heart murmurs
- Previous Kawasaki's disease or rheumatic fever without valvular dysfunction
- Cardiac pacemakers and implanted defibrillators

Modified from Dajani AS, Bisno AL, Chung KJ, et al. Prevention of bacterial endocarditis: Recommendations of the American Heart Association. JAMA 264:2919–2922, 1990.

Table 1–5. CONDITIONS IN OBSTETRICS AND GYNECOLOGY THAT REQUIRE PROPHYLAXIS

Prophylaxis Recommended
- Dental procedures known to produce gingival or mucosal bleeding
- Urethral dilation
- Urethral catheterization or urinary tract surgery if infection present
- Incision and drainage of infected tissue
- Vaginal hysterectomy
- Vaginal delivery with chorioamnionitis

Prophylaxis Not Recommended
- Dental procedures not associated with bleeding
- Injection of local intraoral anesthetic
- Shedding of primary teeth
- Endotracheal intubation
- Cesarean section
- In the absence of infection for urethral catheterization, dilation and curettage, uncomplicated vaginal delivery, abortion, sterilization procedures, or insertion or removal of intrauterine devices

Modified from Dajani AS, Bisno AL, Chung KJ, et al. Prevention of bacterial endocarditis: Recommendations of the American Heart Association. JAMA 264:2919–2922, 1990.

Severe postoperative hypertensive crises are usually treated by infusions of nitroglycerin or nitroprusside. Patients with suspected hypovolemia should be fluid resuscitated prior to initiation of antihypertensive therapy, or severe hypotension may result. Owing to the potency of these agents, an arterial line should be placed and the intensive care unit utilized.

Pulmonary

Theophylline, beta-2 aerosols (albuterol, metaproterenol), and steroids are common therapeutic agents in the treatment of bronchospastic disease. Patients receiving chronic theophylline should remain on these derivatives during the postoperative time period. Because dosage schedules vary as a result of age, cigarette smoking, and drug interactions (cimetidine, erythromycin), an internist should be consulted. Patients who are on constant infusion of theophylline should be monitored daily with serum levels to prevent toxicity. Beta-2 aerosols should be continued in the pre- and postoperative period.

Steroid use of greater than 7.5 mg per day of prednisone for more than 1 week in the prior year requires steroid replacement in the perioperative time period. Additionally, those patients who become bronchospastic either during surgery or postoperatively will also require steroids. A convenient scheme for replacement is: 100 mg hydrocortisone acetate 1 hour prior to surgery, then 100 mg every 8 hours for the first 24 hours. On the second day,

reduce the schedule to 100 mg every 12 hours followed by a single morning dose. On the remaining days, begin 20 mg of prednisone on the first day of oral medication and then reduce by 5 mg of prednisone per day until the patient is on the original chronic dosage prior to surgery. If the patient has discontinued chronic steroids 4 weeks or longer prior to surgery, they can be discontinued after 1 day of 5 mg.

If re-exploration is necessary or the patient becomes septic, restart from the day 1 regimen and taper as outlined above. High doses (hydrocortisone, 100 mg every 6 to 8 hours) should be continued until the patient either has responded to sepsis treatment or is improving after exploration.

Mechanical ventilation in the postoperative period is usually necessary in patients who have a long history of COPD, characterized by a FEV_1 of less than 600 ml. Additional candidates for postoperative mechanical ventilation include elderly patients who undergo prolonged surgery.

Gastrointestinal

Preoperative planning includes an assessment of whether the possibility of bowel surgery exists and if the gastrointestinal tract will require preparation. Proper preparation of the bowel should prevent spillage of formed bowel contents into the peritoneal cavity and therefore reduces the risk of infection and the need for a colostomy. The mechanisms for adequate bowel preparation are often based on the individual surgeon's preference. The most efficacious bowel preparation should involve minimal patient intolerance and physiologic alterations. Table 1–6 reviews a standard bowel preparation that is simple and efficacious.

Endocrinology

In hypothyroid patients, thyroid replacement should be restarted within 3 to 4 days of surgery. Intravenous preparations are available if the patient cannot tolerate oral administration. If the patient is severely hypothyroid, surgery can usually be safely performed, but only on an emergency basis. In patients who require thyroid replacement and have underlying cardiac disease, the initiation of therapy should be started at extremely low levels (0.025 mg of levothyroxin) to avoid myocardial ischemia. Duration of therapy until the euthyroid state is reached usually requires 4 to 6 weeks of therapy.

The thyrotoxic patient who requires emergency

Table 1–6. SCHEME FOR PREOPERATIVE BOWEL PREPARATION

Morning Prior to Surgery
• Mix Golytely* solution and refrigerate

Early Afternoon Prior to Surgery
• 4 liters administered either orally or via a nasogastric tube over 3 hours (20–30 ml/min or 1.3 liters/hr)
• Diarrhea usually begins within 40 minutes
• Rectal effluent clears within 3 hours

Evening of Surgery (optional for elderly and admitted patients)
• Begin intravenous fluids (5% dextrose with ½ normal saline with 20 mEq of potassium chloride) at 75 to 125 ml/hr (lower infusion rate in the elderly and in patients with left ventricular dysfunction)

Morning of Surgery
• Begin intravenous fluids if not previously started
• Administer antibiotics parenterally prior to induction of anesthesia
• Antibiotic regimens (suggested)
Third-generation cephalosprorin (cefotaxime, ceftizoxime) with either clindamycin 600 mg, or metronidazole 500 mg.

*Braintree Laboratories, Inc., Braintree, MA.

surgery should be treated with beta blockers (propranolol 40 mg twice a day), propylthiouracil (300 mg four times a day), and glucocorticoids (hydrocortisone acetate 100 mg every 8 hours) to inhibit transformation of T_4 to T_3 in body tissues. Intravenous iodine (1 g of NaI_2 intravenously) or saturated solution of potassium iodide (SSKI) is given acutely to impede thyroxine release from the thyroid gland. Patients should be initially stabilized for approximately 6 to 12 hours prior to initiation of surgery. If surgery is not acutely needed, stabilization over a period of 3 to 4 weeks is indicated.

Multiple regimens for the dosing of insulin in the insulin-dependent diabetes mellitus (IDDM, or Type I) patient have been championed. The easiest and most effective way is to administer insulin by constant infusion. An infusion of approximately 1 to 1½ units per hour should be given to the patient concurrently with dextrose-containing solutions. Most anesthesiologists prefer to maintain the patient in a slightly hyperglycemic state (150 to 225 mg/dl) intraoperatively secondary to the loss of normal defense mechanisms from hypoglycemia (most anesthetic agents are adrenolytic). The IDDM patient should **never** have insulin infusion discontinued for hypoglycemia but should have a glucose infusion increased with a decrease in insulin infusion (0.5 unit/hour). After surgery, euglycemia should be obtained to decrease wound and infectious complications.

The non–insulin-dependent diabetic (NIDDM, or Type II) usually can be rendered euglycemic by diet within 24 hours. Few of these patients will require insulin once diet is modified. Some patients, however, will become acidotic during the surgery from stress and/or infection. Treatment guidelines are the same as for the IDDM patient, and a constant insulin infusion is initiated until the patient's condition stabilizes for 24 to 48 hours. NIDDM patients may require additional fluids intra- and postoperatively from an osmotic diuresis induced by hyperglycemia.

Diabetics should be closely monitored for signs of impending diabetic ketoacidosis (DKA). An increased respiratory rate may signal the early compensatory respiratory alkalosis stage of an underlying metabolic acidosis. Bedside glucometers are useful to monitor blood sugars, and sampling should be performed at least 4 times a day until the patient stabilizes. Electrolytes should be monitored daily (until the patient is on a regular diet) for a decrease in serum bicarbonate, another indication of early stages of DKA.

Renal and Fluid Requirements

Fluid status is probably the single most important variable in the surgical patient. If replacement of fluids is inadequate, hypoperfusion of vascular beds, acidosis, and shock may intervene. Owing to the necessity of replacing blood loss and losses of fluids from third spacing, adjunctive fluids are necessary. Most fluid requirements are met with either normal saline or Ringer's lactate. Infusion rates vary owing to the state of preoperative hydration, age, and intraoperative blood loss. Postoperative fluid requirements also vary as a result of third spacing of fluid, especially when preoperative ascites is present from ovarian cancer. The elderly patient requires less fluid owing to decreased body mass and may easily become fluid-overloaded. Additionally, the elderly patient may have left ventricular compromise and will not withstand rapid fluid challenges.

The average fluid maintenance for an adult is 125 ml per hour. Normal blood loss is replaced with 3 ml of crystalloid for every 1 ml of blood loss. For the patient who has received a bowel prep or is a poorly controlled diabetic (osmotic diuresis), increased quantities of fluid may be necessary. Third-space fluid losses secondary to intra-abdominal manipulations may lead to additional fluid needs in the first 24 hours in order to maintain intravascular volume. Oliguria, however, may be the first sign of occult bleeding, and other vital signs should be closely monitored. Extensive peritoneal disease, whether it be infectious or carcinoma, may increase third spacing and require increased fluids. The use of diuretics in the postoperative period, except to treat congestive heart failure, should be discouraged. In the patient who becomes intensely oliguric without obvious changes in vital signs, frequent measurements of hematocrit are necessary to rule out occult intra-abdominal bleeding. In cases where the hematocrit remains stable, increased fluids should be used. Except in the elderly patient, fluid challenges of 250 to 500 cc can be given every 15 to 30 minutes.

If prolonged hypotension occurs during surgery, the possibility of acute tubular necrosis should be entertained and large fluid boluses discouraged. When fluid balance is unknown, especially in the patient with renal insufficiency or congestive heart failure, a pulmonary artery catheter may be indicated. Prior to this, pulse oximetry, as well as an arterial blood gas level, should be obtained to rule out hypoxia, especially from congestive heart failure.

Renal insufficiency, or renal failure, necessitates the need for close fluid monitoring. Dialysis patients usually undergo dialysis on the day prior to surgery and on the first postoperative day. Use of a pulmonary artery catheter should be planned in patients who are undergoing extensive dissections or when large blood loss is possible (greater than 1000 ml). Central venous access should be considered preoperatively, except in relatively short procedures. Lastly, hypertension in this group of patients may be a sign of volume overload.

Patients who have undergone extensive bowel preps or who require prolonged nasogastric suctioning will need potassium supplementation. Bowel contents lost during bowel preps reflect colonic losses of potassium and bicarbonate. Prolonged nasogastric (NG) suction results in losses of hydrogen chloride and potassium. To compensate for NG losses, replacement strategies are usually to replace NG losses with an equivalent amount of normal saline with 20 mEq of potassium. Patients with renal failure should have their serum potassium monitored closely, and replacement solutions should not contain more than 10 mEq unless indicated. Frequent monitoring of levels of electrolytes, creatinine, blood urea nitrogen, and potassium should be performed in patients with renal failure.

Postoperative Pain Management

Postoperative pain management has undergone numerous changes in the past 15 years. Intermittent intramuscular narcotic use has decreased with the introduction of constant infusion techniques. Patient-controlled analgesia (PCA) allows the physician to set a constant rate of analgesic (1 mg of morphine per hour) supplemented by intermittent boluses by the patient (1 mg of morphine every 10 minutes). A smaller quantity of a single narcotic is used over a period of time, and patients report better pain control. In the patient with pulmonary disorders, use of PCA contributes to less respiratory depression and therefore less atelectasis and subsequent pneumonias. Additionally, ambulation can be started earlier.

Transcutaneous patches have been developed to deliver a continuous rate of analgesics. The major limitation is the necessary time needed for these drugs to be effective (currently 10 to 12 hours). In the initial postoperative phase, these patches should be used with PCA pumps. PCA pumps should be adjusted to lower doses of medication and discontinued after 12 hours.

Epidural catheters are used to administer long-acting narcotic derivatives. When used as an adjunct with general anesthesia, less systemic agents are administered, and medications can be given through the catheter for postoperative analgesia. These techniques may be helpful in the patient with compromised myocardial function. The elderly patient has a decreased pain threshold and is more sensitive to narcotic agents. The use of the epidural catheter may be especially suited for this group. Many of these patients may require no more than parenteral doses of diphenhydramine HCl, supplemented with low doses of morphine derivatives in the early postoperative period.

Prophylaxis for Deep Venous Thrombosis

A serious, mostly preventable, complication of surgery is deep vein thrombosis (DVT). Risk assessment for DVT is becoming important to selected patients who will benefit from therapy. Mechanical compression with surgical stockings, early ambulation, and pharmacologic manipulations using heparin and Coumadin are standard methods that are in common use. A new device, the sequential compression device (SCD), has become popular in recent years. This device mimics the alternating contractions of leg muscles and increases venous flows. The use of various therapies is usually based on the surgeon's experience.

Factors that significantly increase the potential of thrombosis include (1) older age, especially over the age of 50; (2) anticipated confinement to bed longer than 72 hours; (3) prior history of DVT, pulmonary embolism, or stroke; (4) obesity; (5) left ventricular dysfunction (history of congestive heart failure or pulmonary edema); (6) planned operation in excess of 2 hours; (7) malignancy; (8) pregnancy; and (9) history of hypercoagulable state.

Early ambulation should be attempted in all patients who are not confined to bedrest by pre-existing medical conditions or who require prolonged intensive care unit support in the postoperative period. Patients who are at significant risk are usually treated with a combination of pharmaceutical agents and SCD. The usual dose of heparin is 5000 units subcutaneously every 12 hours, begun 2 hours prior to surgery and discontinued when the patient is fully ambulatory (48 to 72 hours). If the patient is significantly obese (more than 120 per cent of ideal body weight or over 100 kg), the dose of heparin is increased to 7500 units every 12 hours. In our institution, we have opted to discontinue Coumadin and convert the patient to subcutaneous heparin in the above doses in the perioperative period (12 hours prior and post surgery). After the first 12 hours postoperatively, we change from intermittent injection to a constant infusion of heparin (100 units/kg loading dose followed by infusion of 15 units/kg/hour). Heparin is continued at these doses even when Coumadin is begun on the third postoperative day until adequate anticoagulation (measured by the prothrombin time) is reached.

Venous Access for Long-term Therapy

Major advances in nutritional therapy and chemotherapy have had an impact on long-term salvage and survival in many patients. Reliable long-term venous access is necessary to implement these therapies. Multiple devices have been introduced; however, many concepts remain constant in their use. First, many are placed in the subclavian vein because of the lack of mobility in this area, in contrast to an internal jugular approach. Second, the skin entrance is distant to vein catheterization and is tunneled through the subcutaneous tissue to minimize infectious complications. Third, the internal diameter of the catheter should be large enough for ease of infusion and for blood drawing. Lastly, the patient should be able to dress and clean the area after instruction. Several commercial kits are available and should be individualized for specific patient needs. The current technique for placement of a long-dwelling catheter is explained in the legends (Groshong or Lifeport catheter placement). The subclavian approach for central venous access should be reviewed prior to placement (see Figures 1–10 to 1–23).

SUMMARY

Major advances in medical management have contributed to improved outcome, especially in patients compromised by chronic medical ailments. Preoperative work-ups, appropriate consultation, and a well-coordinated team approach have a beneficial role in surgical outcome. A systematic evaluation of each major organ system and perioperative management plan should be implemented prior to

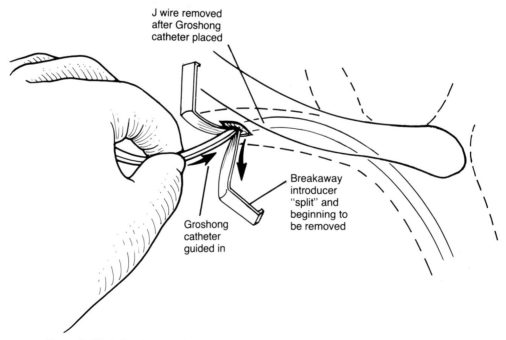

Figure 1-19. A Groshong catheter is threaded through the breakaway catheter.

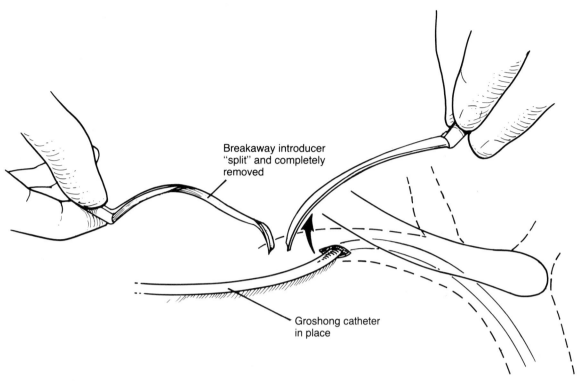

Breakaway introducer "split" and completely removed

Groshong catheter in place

Figure 1-20. The breakaway catheter is withdrawn, split its entire length, and removed.

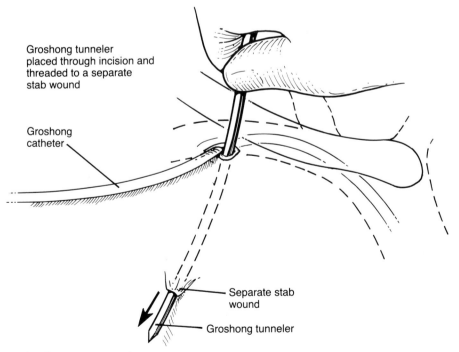

Groshong tunneler placed through incision and threaded to a separate stab wound

Groshong catheter

Separate stab wound

Groshong tunneler

Figure 1-21. A large spike-like device (the Groshong tunneler) is pushed inferiorly through the original incision approximately 5 to 8 cm, creating a separate stab wound. The distal end of the catheter is attached to the tunneler.

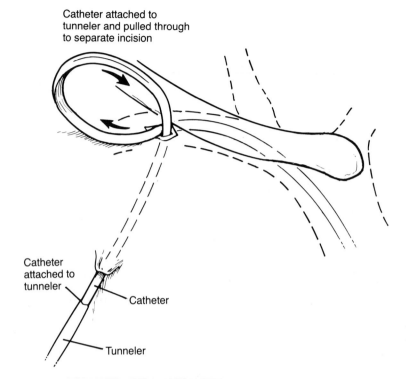

Catheter attached to
tunneler and pulled through
to separate incision

Catheter
attached to
tunneler

Catheter

Tunneler

Figure 1-22. The Groshong catheter is pulled through the separate stab wound and removed from the tunneling device. A permanent cap is placed on the proximal catheter end, and heparin flush is infused.

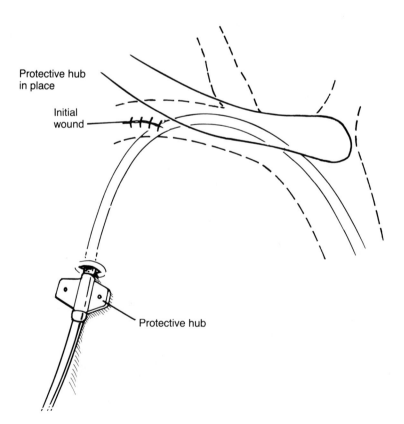

Protective hub
in place

Initial
wound

Protective hub

Figure 1-23. Final closure. The initial wound is closed with 4-0 polyglycolic acid, either with interrupted sutures (as shown) or in a subcutaneous fashion with additional adhesive strips as needed. The distal stab wound is stabilized by suturing a protective hub in place. The hub is removed in 3 weeks, when the entry site has healed. If a Lifeport or other permanent subcutaneous devices are used, a pocket is created. The port is sutured to the fascia. The catheter is attached to the port, and the incision is closed.

the actual surgical event. The use of advanced technology should be considered after carefully weighing the potential risks and benefits. Overall morbidity and mortality should continue to fall with these measures.

REFERENCES

1. Byyny RL: Preventing adrenal insufficiency during surgery. Postgrad Med 65:219–228, 1980.
2. Dajani AS, Bisno AL, Chung KJ, et al: Prevention of bacterial endocarditis: Recommendations by the American Heart Association. JAMA 264:2919–2922, 1990.
3. Detsky AS, Abrams HB, Forbath N, et al: Cardiac assessment for patients undergoing noncardiac surgery. A multifactorial clinical risk index. Arch Intern Med 146:2131–2134, 1986.
4. Fleites RA, Marshall JB, Eekhauser ML, et al: The efficacy of polyethylene glycol–electrolyte lavage solution versus traditional mechanical bowel preparation for elective colonic surgery: A randomized, prospective, blinded clinical trial. Surgery 98:708–717, 1985.
5. Gerson MC, Hurst JM, Hertzberg VS: Cardiac prognosis in noncardiac geriatric surgery. Ann Intern Med 103:832–837, 1985.
6. Goldman L: Cardiac risks and complications of noncardiac surgery. Ann Intern Med 98:504–513, 1983.
7. Goldman L, Caldera D: Risks of general anesthesia and elective operative in the hypertensive patient. Anesthesiology 50:285–292, 1979.
8. Goldman L, Caldera DL, Southwich FS, et al: Cardiac risk factors and complications in non-cardiac surgery. Medicine 57:357–370, 1978.
9. Keating HJ: Perioperative considerations in the geriatric patient. Med Clin North Am 71:569–583, 1987.
10. McMurry JF Jr: Wound healing with diabetes mellitus: Better glucose control for better wound healing in diabetes. Surg Clin North Am 64:769–778, 1984.
11. Nolan TE, Wakefield ML, Devoe LD: Invasive hemodynamic monitoring in obstetrics: A critical review of its indications, benefits, complications, and alternatives. Chest 101:1429–1433, 1992.
12. Pasulka PS, Bistrian BR, Benotti PN, Glackburn GL: The risks of surgery in obese patients. Ann Intern Med 104:540–546, 1986.
13. Tisi GM: Preoperative identification and evaluation of the patient with lung disease. Med Clin North Am 71:399–412, 1987.
14. Torrington KG, Henderson CJ: Perioperative respiratory therapy (PORT): A program of preoperative risk assessment and individualized postoperative care. Chest 93:946–951, 1988.

2

Alternate Surgical Procedures for Early Vulvar Carcinoma

The traditional treatment for invasive squamous carcinoma of the vulva has been en bloc radical vulvectomy and bilateral groin lymph node dissection. This groin dissection included both the superficial and deep inguinal nodes. Following the description by Byron and associates[3] of vulvectomy and bilateral groin dissection using three separate incisions, several authors have described excellent survival and much reduced postoperative complications when the three incision technique was used. Following a report from the M. D. Anderson Hospital and Tumor Institute concerning limited surgery for "microinvasive" carcinoma of the vulva, DiSaia and colleagues[4] and others have suggested a more limited approach for early stage carcinoma of the vulva. Because of the metastatic pattern of invasive vulvar carcinoma from the superficial to the deep inguinal nodes, the superficial groin nodes are felt to be the sentinel nodes for vulvar malignancies. A yet unpublished study by the Gynecologic Oncology Group suggests that the procedure described below can be a safe alternative in *carefully selected* patients. More young women are presenting with invasive vulvar lesions, and the gynecologist is faced with the challenge of achieving a high cure rate while limiting anatomic dysformity and preserving psychosexual function.

Generally, the limited resection described below is indicated only in patients with T1 lesions (2 cm or less in size). The histologic evaluation of an excisional biopsy should reveal no tumor invading more than 5 mm measured from the surface. Furthermore, capillary and lymphatic space involvement should not be noted in the excised specimen. For lateral lesions, an ipsilateral superficial groin lymph node dissection should be done. However, for central lesions, a bilateral superficial groin lymph node dissection should be performed. A frozen section of the superficial nodes should be obtained. If any nodes are positive, the deep nodes should be removed and a more radical excision of the involved vulva performed.

Pathophysiologic changes from this operation are later accumulation of lymph tissue and lymphangitis in a small percentage of patients. In order to avoid the problem of lymph accumulation, the inferior lymphatic bundles should be clamped and suture ligated.

POTENTIAL PROBLEM AREAS

In addition to the accumulation of lymph fluid when the inferior lymph tissue is not ligated, injury to the saphenous vein in thin patients is a possibility. This is more likely to occur if the dissection is carried posterior to the cribriform fascia. In order to avoid later wound breakdown, it is always wise to carefully inspect the wound edges. If there is any question about the viability of the edges, the skin edges should be freshened by removing a small amount of skin and subcutaneous tissue on the superior and inferior borders. Closed suction drainage will also help avoid the problem with later accumulation of lymph fluid.

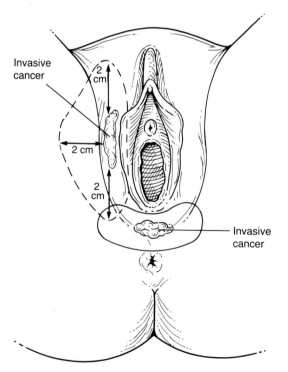

Figure 2–1. Small primary carcinomas are shown on the right labia majora in the perineum. The wide local excision should generally include a 1- to 2-cm margin. A generous amount of subcutaneous tissue should be removed because this is an invasive lesion. Many patients will have had a previous excisional biopsy, and a 2-cm margin around the prior scar should be maintained.

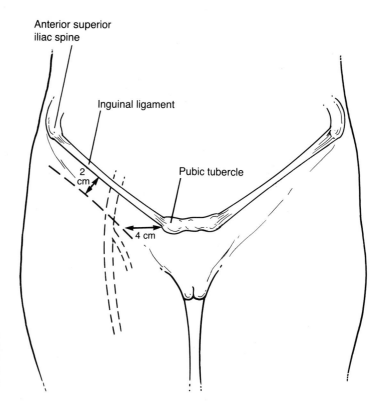

Figure 2–2. A groin incision approximately 8 cm in length will suffice for most patients. The incision is made 4 cm lateral to the pubic tubercle and 2 cm below, but parallel to, the inguinal ligament. Thus, the incision should be in the general area of the fossa ovalis and of the saphenofemoral junction.

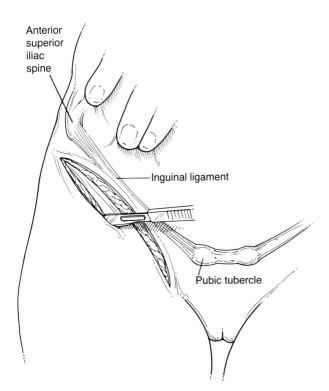

Figure 2–3. We prefer to preserve a wedge of skin tissue to grasp the bundle with Allis clamps to exert proper countertraction. The incision is carried down to the level of Camper's fascia.

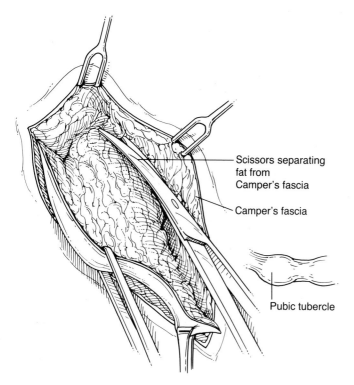

Scissors separating
fat from
Camper's fascia

Camper's fascia

Pubic tubercle

Figure 2–4. Skin hooks are placed on Camper's fascia. Using sharp dissection, a plane is developed beneath the fascia. Blunt dissection with a knife handle can also be used to develop this plane just below Camper's fascia. Countertraction with Allis clamps is maintained on the specimen. Once the superior mobilization has been done, the inferior tissue is mobilized in a similar manner.

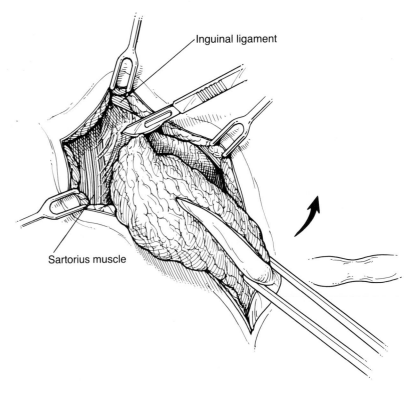

Inguinal ligament

Sartorius muscle

Figure 2–5. Once the subcutaneous tissue containing the sentinel nodes is mobilized cephalad and caudad by sharp and blunt dissection, the incision is carried out on the lateral border down to the fascia overlying the sartorius muscle. The bundle of tissue is then mobilized from lateral to medial by sharp and blunt dissection. To avoid later accumulation of lymph fluid, the inferior lymphatic tissue should be clamped and suture ligated.

Figure 2–6. The cribriform fascia is the inferior border of dissection. It fuses and is continuous with the fascia lata of the thigh. The tissue should be mobilized superior to the level of the inguinal ligament and inferiorly to the level approximately 2 cm cephalad to the beginning of Hunter's canal. In some thin patients, a plane of the cribriform fascia is not usually maintained. The saphenous vein is encountered just medial and slightly anterior to the femoral artery and femoral vein. It lies posterior to the cribriform fascia. If there is a question as to its position, it should be isolated as shown here with a vessel loop. Perforating vessels should be isolated for later ligation. They should be individually tied or clipped.

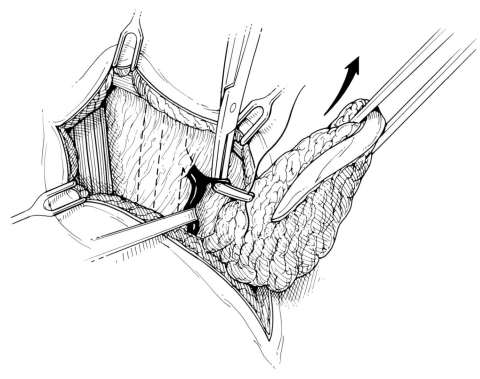

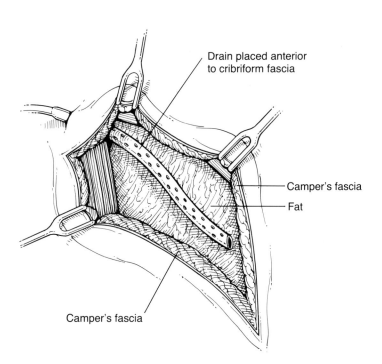

Drain placed anterior to cribriform fascia

Camper's fascia

Fat

Camper's fascia

Figure 2–7. Following removal of the tissue bundle containing the sentinel nodes, it is sent for frozen section. If metastatic disease is found in any of the nodes, a deep inguinal node dissection should be performed. A flat Jackson-Pratt or Blake drain is placed anterior to the cribriform fascia and brought out through a stab wound lateral to the incision.

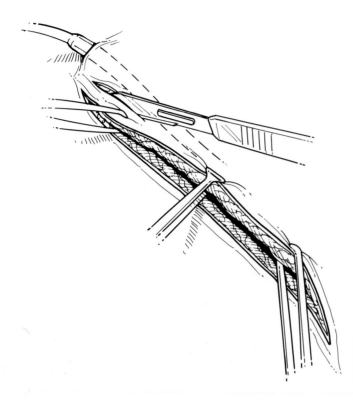

Figure 2–8. If the wound edges appear compromised, a 5-mm to 1-cm strip of skin is excised by using Allis clamps for counter-traction. After the superior wound edge is freshened as shown, the inferior edge can be managed in a similar manner.

Figure 2–9. Interrupted sutures of 3-0 polyglycolic acid are used to reunite the edges of Camper's fascia over the drain. The skin can be closed with staples as shown, with mattress sutures of nylon or monofilament polypropylene, or with sub-cuticular polyglycolic acid suture, depending on the patient's abdominal wall thickness. If the three-incision technique is used for T2 lesions or for more invasive vulvar carcinoma, the separate groin incisions can be made as described. The deep groin nodes can be removed en bloc or separately. Surgical excision of the vulvar lesion should be made and tailored on an individualized basis.

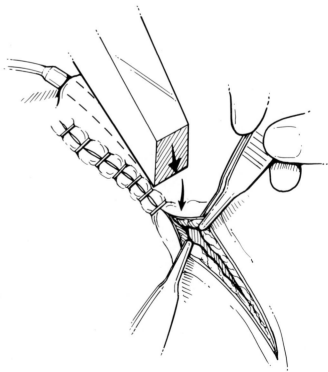

REFERENCES

1. Ballon SC, Lamb EJ: Separate incisions in the treatment of carcinoma of the vulva. Surg Gynecol Obstet 140:81–87, 1975.
2. Burke TW, Stringer A, Gershenson DM, et al: Radical wide excision and selective inguinal node dissection for squamous cell carcinoma of the vulva. Gynecol Oncol 38:328, 1990.
3. Byron RL, Lamb EJ, Yonemoto RH, et al: Radical inguinal node dissection in the treatment of cancer. Surg Gynecol Obstet 114:401–411, 1962.
4. DiSaia PJ, Creasman WT, Rich WM: An alternate approach to early cancer of the vulva. Am J Obstet Gynecol 133:825–832, 1979.
5. Hacker NF, Leuchter RS, Berek JS, et al: Radical vulvectomy and bilateral inguinal lymphadenectomy through separate groin incisions. Obstet Gynecol 58:574–578, 1981.
6. Hacker NF, Berek JS, Lagasse LD, et al: Individualization of treatment for stage I squamous cell vulvar carcinoma. Obstet Gynecol 63:155, 1984.
7. Hacker NF: Current treatment of small vulvar cancers. Oncology 4:21, 1990.
8. Sutton GP, Miser MR, Stehman FS, et al: Trends in operative management of invasive squamous carcinoma of the vulva at Indiana University, 1974 to 1988. Am J Obstet Gynecol 164:1472, 1991.
9. Wilkinson EJ, Rico MJ, Pierson KK: Microinvasive carcinoma of the vulva. Int J Gynaecol Pathol 1:29, 1982.

3

Radical Vulvectomy and Groin Dissection

Treatment of invasive cancer of the vulva is primarily surgical. The classic operation—en bloc removal of vulva and groin nodes—has been challenged in favor of lesser procedures, depending on individual circumstances. Nevertheless, its inclusion in any surgical atlas is mandatory, because it represents the gold standard to which the lesser procedures are compared for end results.

The peak incidence of vulvar cancer is in the sixth and seventh decades of life; thus, detection and evaluation of chronic underlying processes, e.g., hypertension, diabetes, arteriosclerosis, etc., is an integral part of the work-up in these patients. Local evaluation includes a proper clinical staging: size of the lesion, involvement of adjacent structures (e.g., urethra, vagina, anus), and clinical status of lymph nodes (FIGO TNM classification). Ancillary tests include cystoscopy, proctosigmoidoscopy, and computed tomography scan of the abdomen and pelvis in selected patients.

This chapter illustrates the "classic" en bloc dissection of vulva and groin.

The bowel is cleansed with one of the available bowel prep protocols. A central line (triple lumen) is inserted the night before or at surgery.

PATHOPHYSIOLOGIC CHANGES

Patients need ample time for counseling prior to surgery. The operation as described denotes a "change in body image" with its psychosexual implications. Other changes depend on the extension of the resection, e.g., urinary incontinence following partial resection of the urethra, dyspareunia due to scarring and stenosis of the introitus, and partial fecal incontinence due to damage to the sphincteric mechanism or nerve supply when resecting perineal and perianal lesions. With the advent of modified or partial vulvectomies, the majority of changes have been largely eliminated.

POTENTIAL RISKS

Operative deep dissection of the groin can result in injury to the femoral vessels and nerves. When performing deep groin dissection, transplantation of the sartorius muscle should be done to prevent trauma to the unprotected vessels.

POSTOPERATIVE CARE

An indwelling bladder catheter is kept in for 4 to 5 days. Oral feeding other than liquids is not permitted for the same period of time. Closed drainage of the groin is continued for as long as the 24-hour suction exceeds 50 ml in each reservoir. On the average, drains remain in place for 10 to 14 days. Drainage is one factor that has significantly improved the primary healing of the groin wounds. Antibiotics to prevent infections of the urinary tract and prophylactic anticoagulants are used routinely.

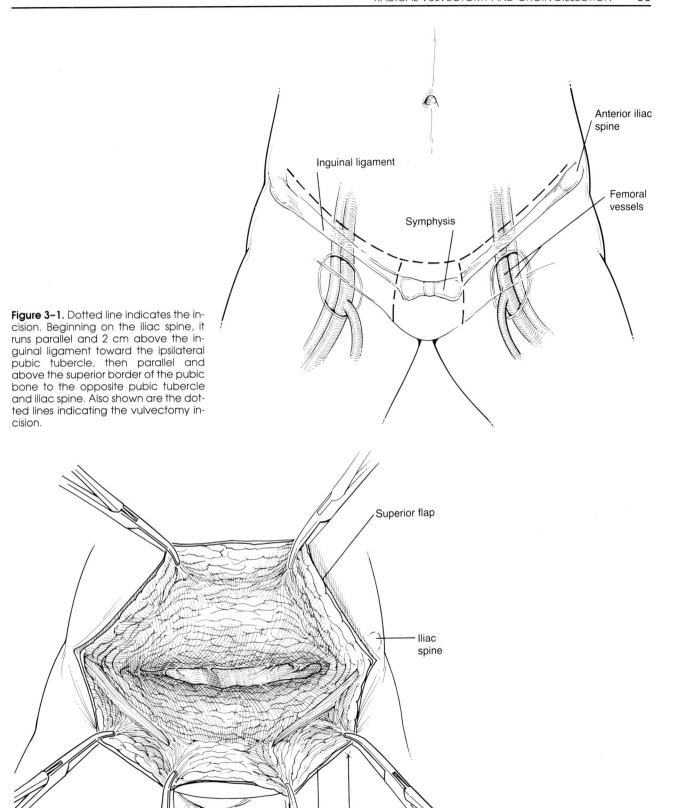

Figure 3–1. Dotted line indicates the incision. Beginning on the iliac spine, it runs parallel and 2 cm above the inguinal ligament toward the ipsilateral pubic tubercle, then parallel and above the superior border of the pubic bone to the opposite pubic tubercle and iliac spine. Also shown are the dotted lines indicating the vulvectomy incision.

Inguinal ligament

Anterior iliac spine

Femoral vessels

Symphysis

Superior flap

Iliac spine

Apex of Scarpa triangle

Inferior flap

Figure 3–2. Superior and inferior flaps are developed, taking care not to skeletonize the skin to prevent flap necrosis. The limits of the superior flap are an imaginary line across the superior iliac spines. The limits of the inferior flaps correspond to the apex of the Scarpa triangles.

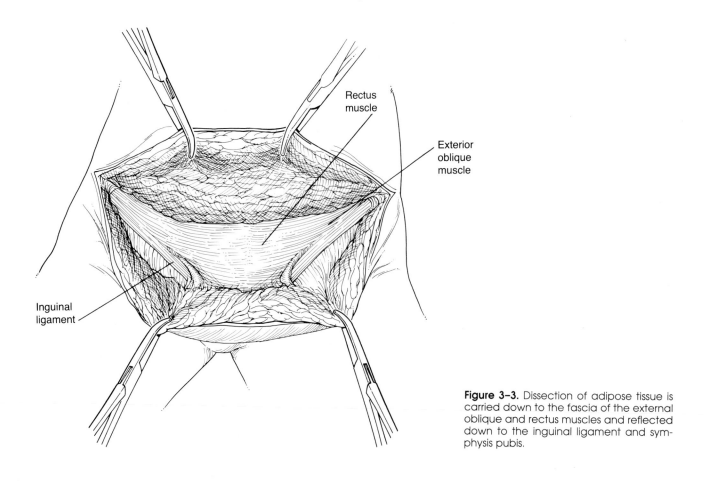

Rectus
muscle

Exterior
oblique
muscle

Inguinal
ligament

Figure 3–3. Dissection of adipose tissue is carried down to the fascia of the external oblique and rectus muscles and reflected down to the inguinal ligament and symphysis pubis.

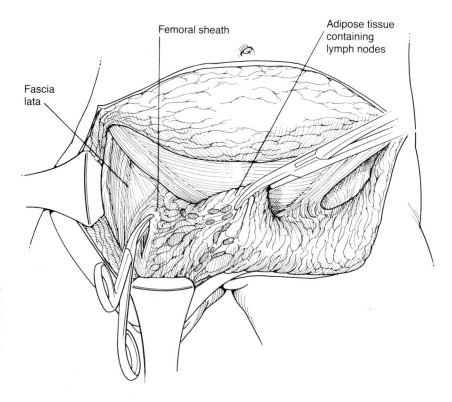

Femoral sheath

Adipose tissue containing lymph nodes

Fascia lata

Figure 3–4. On the inferior flap, dissection is begun laterally and carried down the fascia lata and reflected medially. At the level of the inguinal ligament, lower and upper dissection meet. Dissection continues medially; the femoral sheath is entered, guided by the pulsations of the femoral artery.

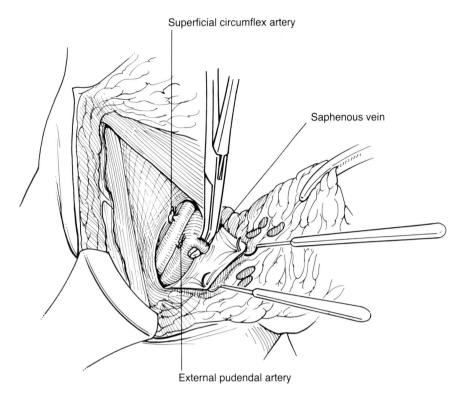

Superficial circumflex artery

Saphenous vein

External pudendal artery

Figure 3–5. Care is taken not to injure the femoral nerve. The artery is dissected down to the apex of the Scarpa triangle. On the medial side, the external pudendal artery is isolated, ligated, and cut. It serves as a consistent landmark for the entry of the saphenous vein on the medial side of the femoral vein. Toward the inguinal ligament, the superficial circumflex artery is found. It can be preserved or sacrificed. The femoral vein is dissected on its external and anterior surface. Having the external pudendal artery as a guide, it is easy to anticipate the entrance of the saphenous vein on its medial side. It is isolated and ligated.

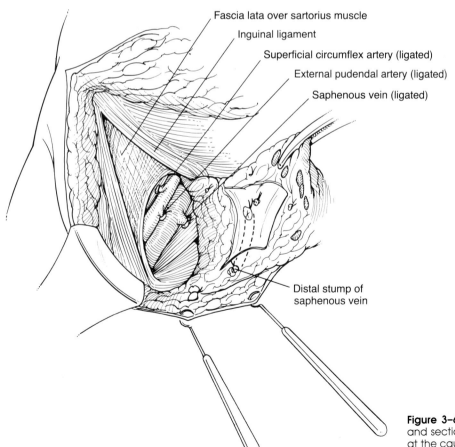

Fascia lata over sartorius muscle

Inguinal ligament

Superficial circumflex artery (ligated)

External pudendal artery (ligated)

Saphenous vein (ligated)

Distal stump of saphenous vein

Figure 3–6. The saphenous vein is also ligated and sectioned on the inner aspect of the thigh at the caudad level of the dissection.

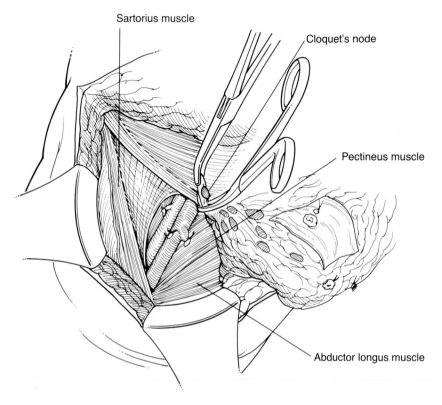

Sartorius muscle

Cloquet's node

Pectineus muscle

Abductor longus muscle

Figure 3–7. Further dissection exposes the fascia of the pectineus muscle. On the proximal and inner aspect of the femoral vein the "Cloquet node" is identified and resected. This node represents the upper limit of the deep groin dissection. If this node is found to be positive, pelvic node dissection may be indicated.

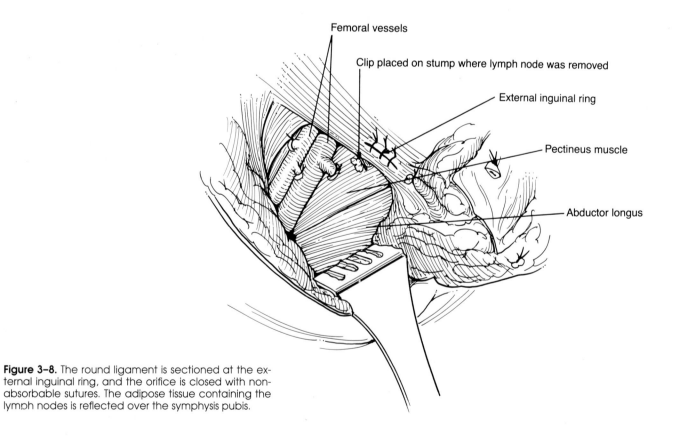

Femoral vessels

Clip placed on stump where lymph node was removed

External inguinal ring

Pectineus muscle

Abductor longus

Figure 3–8. The round ligament is sectioned at the external inguinal ring, and the orifice is closed with nonabsorbable sutures. The adipose tissue containing the lymph nodes is reflected over the symphysis pubis.

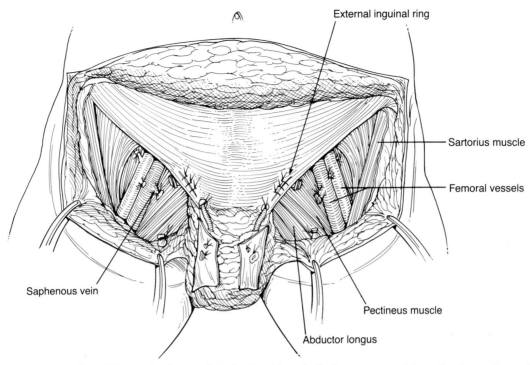

External inguinal ring

Sartorius muscle

Femoral vessels

Saphenous vein

Pectineus muscle

Abductor longus

Figure 3–9. Bilateral dissection of the groins is completed with all lymphatic tissue removed from the femoral vessels and their branches.

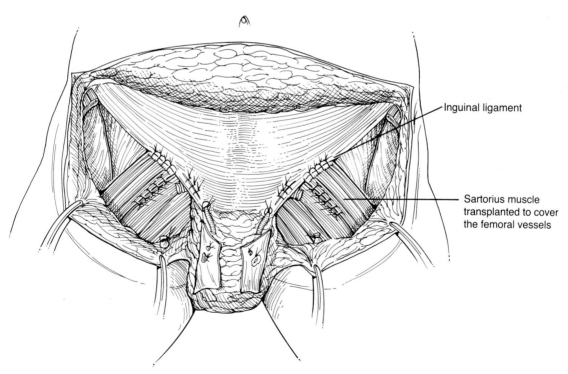

Inguinal ligament

Sartorius muscle transplanted to cover the femoral vessels

Figure 3–10. The fascia lata covering the sartorius muscle is incised, parallel to the muscle, which is dissected cephalad to its attachment at the iliac crest and severed. It is dissected caudad sufficiently to cover the femoral vessels without undue tension. Because its vascular supply is segmented in nature, some branches need to be sacrificed to accomplish adequate mobilization. The muscle and transplanted fascia are attached to the inguinal ligament and pectineal fascia with interrupted sutures of nonabsorbable material.

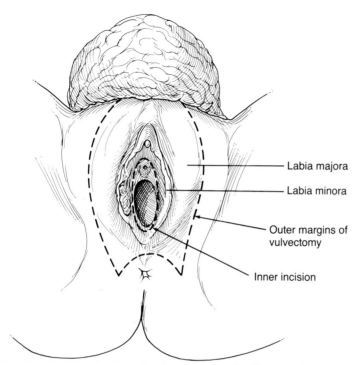

Labia majora

Labia minora

Outer margins of
vulvectomy

Inner incision

Figure 3–11. The area of dissection is loosely packed with moist gauze, and the patient is placed in lithotomy position, simply by elevating the stirrups. The outer excision of the vulvectomy is begun at the mons veneris and extends caudad along the labiocrural folds, encircling the perineum. The inner incision begins just cephalad to the urethral meatus and extends laterally and caudad to encompass all of the vestibule.

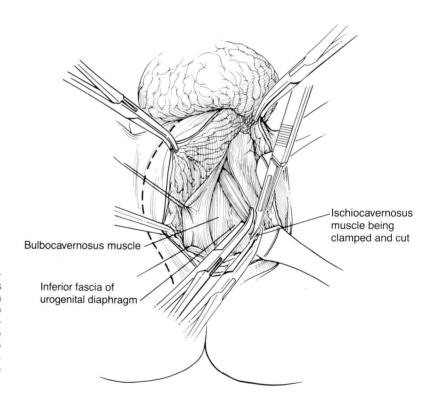

Ischiocavernosus
muscle being
clamped and cut

Bulbocavernosus muscle

Inferior fascia of
urogenital diaphragm

Figure 3–12. Superiorly, the outer incision is carried down to the periosteum of the symphysis pubis; laterally, the superficial perineal pouch is entered by incising Colles fascia in order to remove the ischiocavernosus and bulbo-cavernosus. The limit of the deep dissection is the deep fascia of the urogenital diaphragm. The superficial transverse perineal muscle is not resected, except when perineal lesions are present.

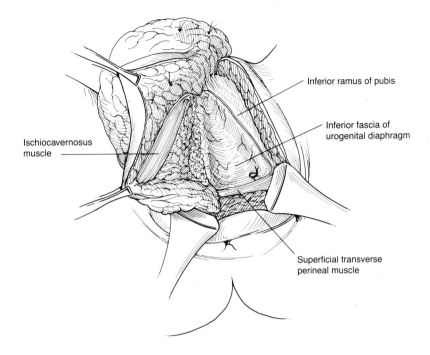

Inferior ramus of pubis

Inferior fascia of urogenital diaphragm

Ischiocavernosus muscle

Superficial transverse perineal muscle

Figure 3–13. A completed dissection of left vulva from symphysis pubis to superficial transverse perineal muscle. At the depth of dissection is the inferior fascia of the urogenital diaphragm. The inner and outer incisions have met at this point.

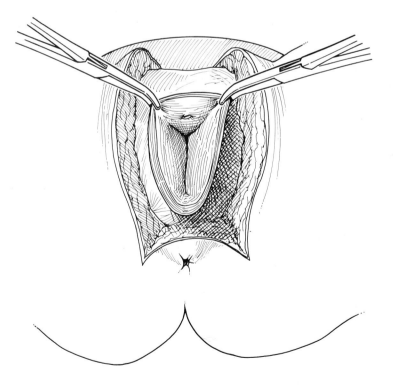

Figure 3–14. The vulvectomy has been performed. The distal vagina is mobilized widely in preparation for closure without undue tension. Note the "butterfly" type of incision perianally. It helps to approximate the perianal skin to the vaginal edges.

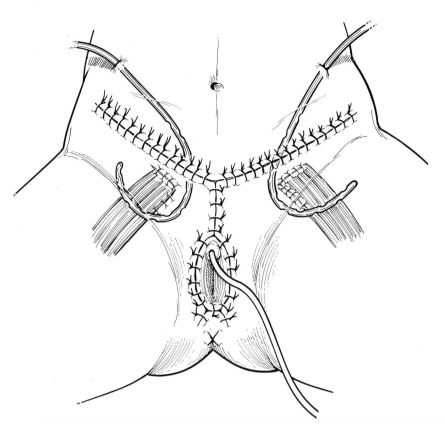

Figure 3–15. The posterior vagina is mobilized widely as for a low posterior repair. A perineoplasty is performed and the vulva and groin areas are approximated. A closed drainage system is utilized on both groins and brought out through stab wounds on the lower quadrants.

REFERENCES

Green TH Jr: Radical vulvectomy. Clin Obstet Gynecol 8:642, 1965.

Parson L, Ulfelder H: An Atlas of Pelvic Surgery. WB Saunders Company, Philadelphia, 1968, pp 350–385.

Thompson JD, Rock JA (eds): TeLinde's Operative Gynecology, 7th ed. JB Lippincott, Philadelphia, 1992, pp 1099–1116.

Wheeless C Jr: Atlas of Pelvic Surgery. Lea and Febiger, Philadelphia, 1981, pp 344–349.

4

Abdominal Incisions and Closures

Abdominal incisions and their closure vary with the urgency for operative intervention, the indications for the operation, and associated preoperative conditions such as presence of ascites or bowel obstruction, suspicion of upper abdominal pathology, and the previous abdominal scar. Incisions for surgery for gynecologic oncology patients should be highly individualized. Incisions should meet certain basic criteria, including reasonably rapid entry, the chance of minimal nerve damage, adequate exposure, and a closure that will leave minimal chance of infection or fascial dehiscence. The need for colostomies, urinary diversions, and extraperitoneal approaches to node-bearing areas must be considered.

The two basic incisions for entrance into the abdominal cavity by the gynecologist performing radical procedures are transverse incisions and their modifications and midline incisions. With the advent of more recent closure methods and newer suture materials, the allegedly stronger paramedian incision is unnecessary.

Transverse incisions offer the advantages of being the best cosmetic incision for pelvic surgery and are less painful, resulting in less interference in pulmonary function. The incision is also made along Langer's lines. Thus, transverse incisions allegedly both are stronger and result in fewer eviscerations than midline incisions. However, eviscerations associated with midline incisions may be due to inappropriate closure techniques. Transverse incisions are more time consuming and may be associated with relatively more bleeding. They are associated with a relative inability to explore the upper abdomen.

Vertical incisions in modern-day gynecologic oncology are basically equated to the midline approach. The midline incision is least hemorrhagic. Rapid entry is feasible. Exposure is excellent, and minimal nerve damage occurs.

In this chapter, incisions related to exploration of the abdominal cavity are outlined. Incisions for such procedures as nodal sampling will be discussed in Chapter 8.

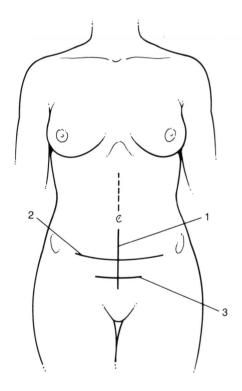

Figure 4-1. For entry into the abdomen, three basic incisions are used: *1*, the midline incision; *2*, the transverse Maylard-type incision from anterior-superior iliac spine to anterior-superior iliac spine, and *3*, the Pfannenstiel incision. This is not an incision for radical pelvic surgery, but its conversion to the Cherney-type incision for better exposure will be shown. For the patient who has some type of transverse incision, and for whom later exposure of the upper abdomen is necessary, a midline upper abdominal incision may be separately used.

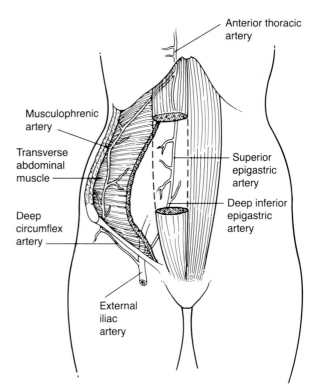

Figure 4–2. The arterial blood supply of the anterior abdominal wall is noted. The deep inferior epigastric artery, which arises from the external iliac artery, is well lateral to the rectus muscle in the caudad portion of the pelvis. Its course gradually runs medially, and it is located on the lateral and posterior border of the rectus muscle. It joins with the superior epigastric artery, which arises from the anterior thoracic artery. Laterally, the deep circumflex iliac arises from the external iliac artery and partially supplies the transverse abdominal muscle. It joins with the musculophrenic artery. When incising the transverse abdominal muscle, the tributaries of these arteries must be watched for. The muscle layers of the anterior abdominal wall will be more thoroughly depicted in Chapter 8.

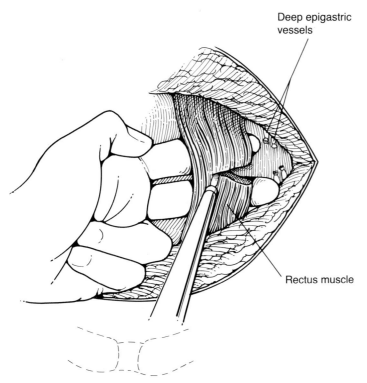

Figure 4–3. The Maylard incision. A transverse incision has been made from the anterior-superior iliac spine to the opposite anterior-superior iliac spine. The fascia has been incised transversely. The deep inferior epigastric vessels are located on the lateral and posterior borders of the rectus muscle. They are bluntly dissected from this position by the finger of the operator, isolated, clamped, sectioned, and tied. Only after they are tied should the rectus muscle be incised. This can be done with the Bovie.

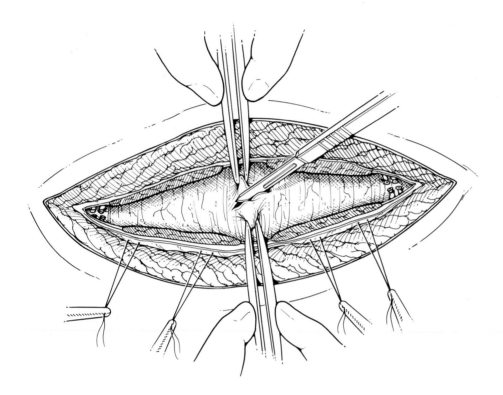

Figure 4–4. The peritoneum is sharply incised with a knife, and the incision is carried transversely. The incision should be well cephalad to the bladder. Note that the vessels have been previously sectioned and tied. The transverse lines (raphe) keep the rectus muscle from retracting. However, we prefer to suture the underlying muscle to the overlying fascia with a 2-0 absorbable suture as noted. The knots should be placed on the fascial side. These sutures are used to ensure hemostasis.

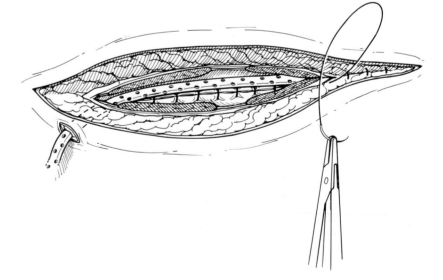

Figure 4–5. The closure of the Maylard incision is done in layers. We suture the peritoneum with a running 3-0 absorbable suture and place a closed drainage system posterior to the fascia and muscle bellies. A No. 1 delayed absorbable suture (Maxon or PDS-2) is used to close the fascia. One suture is started from each end and they are tied in the middle. No attempt is made to reapproximate the rectus muscle bellies.

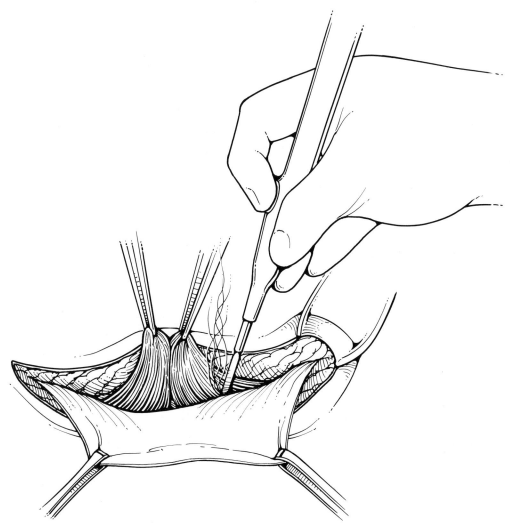

Figure 4–6. The Cherney incision. Occasionally, the pelvic surgeon will make a Pfannenstiel incision and encounter such conditions as a large pelvic mass, severe endometriosis, or lower uterine segment leiomyomata where additional room and exposure are needed. In this situation, the appropriate maneuver is not to half-transect the rectus muscle, because the inferior epigastric vessels may be damaged. The appropriate maneuver is to convert the Pfannenstiel incision to a Cherney. This shows the rectus muscle and pyramidalis being separated from the overlying fascia with the Bovie.

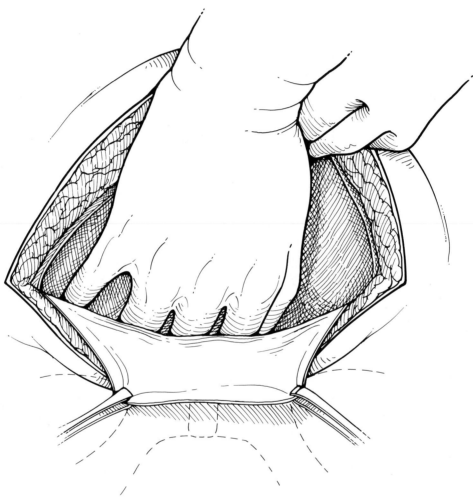

Figure 4–7. The space of Retzius is developed by the weight of the operator's hand gently dissecting the bladder from the overlying symphysis and rectus muscle insertions.

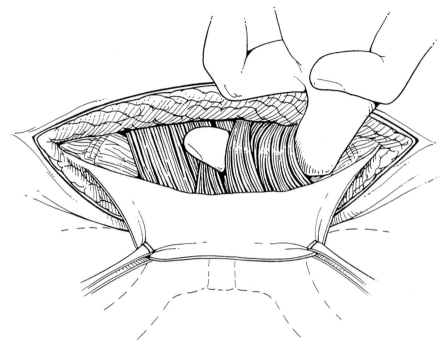

Figure 4-8. The finger of the operator is placed posterior to the rectus muscle, and with gentle traction the muscle is pulled cephalad.

Deep inferior
epigastric vessels

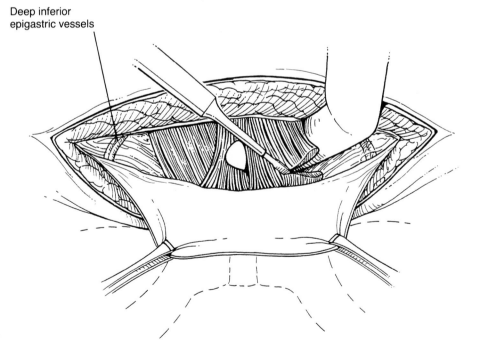

Figure 4-9. With the muscle pulled cephalad, the rectus muscle can be dissected from its insertion at the symphysis by the Bovie. Note the lateral position of the deep inferior epigastric vessels. The peritoneal incision can then be extended laterally, avoiding the deep inferior epigastric vessels.

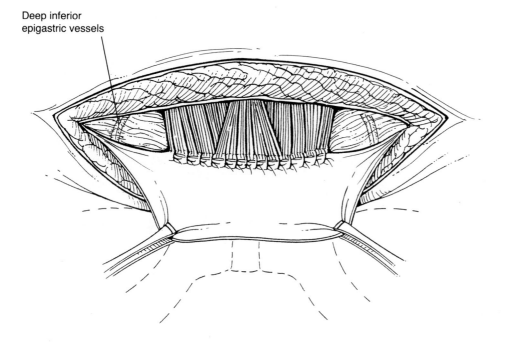

Deep inferior
epigastric vessels

Figure 4-10. The muscles, which include the pyramidalis and rectus, are sutured to the raphe or to the fascia with permanent 2-0 suture. The peritoneum has been previously closed. Note again the lateral position of the deep inferior epigastric vessels. Five to six sutures are used on each side.

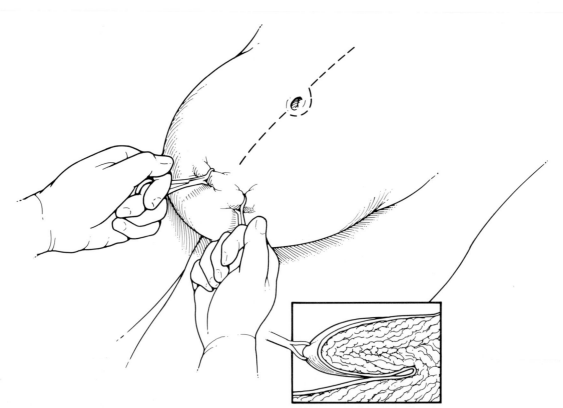

Figure 4-11. The midline incision can be used for any operative procedure in which exposure to the upper abdomen is needed. As shown in this picture, the midline is our preferred incision for the obese patient. This incision becomes a periumbilical incision. The panniculus is drawn inferiorly by Allis clamps or towel clips. Using this maneuver, one avoids making an incision in the anaerobic infested area that lies beneath the subpannicular fold. The midline incision for obese patients is a rapid and relatively bloodless one.

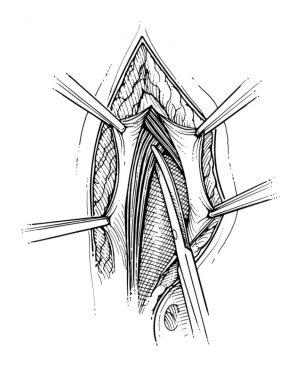

Figure 4-12. Once the muscle bellies have been separated in the midline, the space of Retzius is developed. The raphe between the pyramidalis muscles is sectioned down to the insertion on the symphysis in order to give maximum exposure in the pelvis in obese patients.

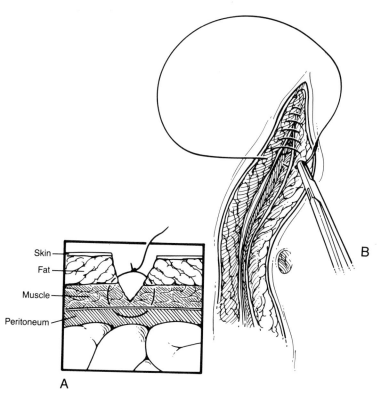

Skin
Fat
Muscle
Peritoneum

A

B

Figure 4-13. A running No. 1 delayed absorbable suture (Maxon or PDS) is used to close midline incisions. We use the Smead-Jones closure only in patients who need re-exploration for fascial dehiscence. One suture is started from the cephalad end, and one is started from the caudad end. The knots are buried. The sutures are placed approximately 1 cm apart. *A,* The sutures are placed at least 2 cm from the fascial edge. The suture bite should include anterior fascia, a portion of the muscle, and the posterior fascia. The peritoneum is included if it is easily located. *B,* When the midpoint is reached from the running suture from cephalad end and caudad end, the sutures are simply tied and the knot buried. Six throws are used for each knot. For obese patients, we prefer to place a closed drainage system (a Blake or Jackson-Pratt) in the subcutaneous space, leaving the drain in for 72 hours or until the drainage is less than 100 ml per day.

REFERENCES

1. Fagniez T, Haye JM, Lacaine F, Thomsen C: Abdominal midline incisions and closure. A randomized prospective trial of 3,135 patients, comparing continuous versus interrupted polyglycolic acid sutures. Arch Surg 120:1351, 1984.
2. Gallup DG, Talledo OE, King LA: Primary mass closure of midline incisions with a continuous running monofilament suture in gynecologic patients. Obstet Gynecol 73:67, 1989.
3. Gallup DG, Nolan TE, Smith RP: Primary mass closure of midline incisions with a continuous polyglyconate monofilament absorbable suture. Obstet Gynecol 76:872, 1990.
4. Jurkiewicz MJ, Morales L: Wound healing, operative incisions, and skin grafts. In Hardy JD: Hardy's Textbook of Surgery. JB Lippincott, Philadelphia, 1983, p 108.
5. Maylard AE: Direction of abdominal incisions. Br Med J 2:895, 1907.
6. Sutton G, Morgan S: Abdominal wound closure using a running, looped monofilament polybustester suture: Comparison to Smead-Jones closure in historic controls. Obstet Gynecol 80:650, 1992.
7. Wallace D, Hernandez W, Schlaerth JB, et al: Prevention of abdominal wound disruption utilizing the Smead-Jones closure technique. Obstet Gynecol 56:226, 1980.

5

Extraperitoneal Pelvic Lymph Node Dissection with Modified Radical Hysterectomy

A modified radical hysterectomy as an alternate surgical treatment for patients with early invasive carcinoma has been advocated by some gynecologic surgeons in order to decrease the operative time and morbidity as compared with the more traditional radical hysterectomy as originally described by Wertheim.[7] In 1974, Piver and associates pointed out the difference between these two procedures and equated the modified radical hysterectomy to a class II and a radical hysterectomy to a class III.[5] In an unrandomized series of patients with stage IB carcinoma of the cervix reported by DiSaia, there was no difference in survival or local recurrences among patients who had a class II versus a class III radical hysterectomy.[1] With a minimal follow-up of 2 years, six cancer deaths occurred in 70 patients who had a class III radical hysterectomy, with three cancer deaths in 40 patients with a class II procedure. Photopulos and Zwagg have shown an expected decrease in ureterovaginal fistulas in a series of patients who underwent modified radical hysterectomy (none) versus those that underwent the traditional radical hysterectomy (three).[4] They also noted a statistically significant decrease in operative time and hospital stay in those undergoing class II hysterectomy. The low incidence of fistula formation with the class II operation is probably due to the lack of dissection of the ureter from the peritoneum, except in the paracervical area. Extrinsic blood supply in the lateral portion of the ureter is sufficient to support the distal portion of the ureter. Generally, the indication for this procedure is in patients who can have the malignancy encompassed by the procedure. Such situations might include patients with conization diagnosis of cervical carcinoma where microinvasion is noted at the cephalad or endocervical margin of the cone. In some institutions, it might include patients with 3 to 5 mm of invasion or patients with capillary-like vascular space involvement in routine sections of a conization. It might be used in carefully selected patients with occult carcinoma of the cervix and in selected cases of gynecologic malignancy following radiation therapy.

Pathophysiologic changes from this operation are minimal. The risk of ureteral or vesicovaginal fistula and bladder atony should be less than with the more radical class III hysterectomy.

POTENTIAL PROBLEM AREAS

We prefer to remove the pelvic nodes extraperitoneally. In the rare case in which significant pelvic metastases are found, survival may be increased by removing these nodes extraperitoneally and proceeding with radiation therapy as reported by Downey and associates.[2] The obturator vessels are in close proximity to the obturator nerve. If they are preserved, their tributaries must be carefully clipped and sectioned prior to removing them from the obturator space. Care must be taken to preserve the blood supply to the lateral portion to the ureter. The ureter, therefore, is not removed from its posterior attachments, but simply rolled laterally in order to obtain a generous amount of parametrium in the resected tissue. Extraperitoneal drainage with a closed drainage system such as a Jackson-Pratt or Blake drain is used for a minimum of 5 days in order to avoid the formation of lymphocysts.

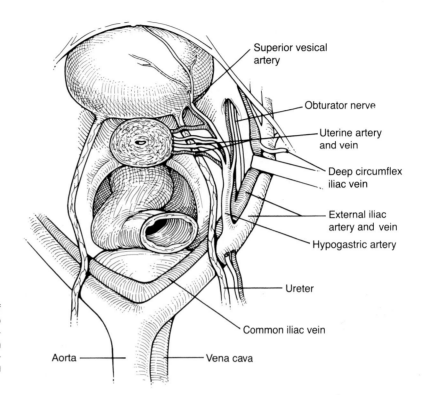

Superior vesical
artery

Obturator nerve

Uterine artery
and vein

Deep circumflex
iliac vein

External iliac
artery and vein

Hypogastric artery

Ureter

Common iliac vein

Aorta   Vena cava

Figure 5-1. Anatomy of major blood vessels of the pelvis. The uterine vessels cross anterior to the ureter. The obturator nerve is located posterior and lateral to the external iliac vein, which has been retracted. Occasionally an anomalous obturator vein will arise from the foramina and enter the external iliac vein.

Space of Retzius

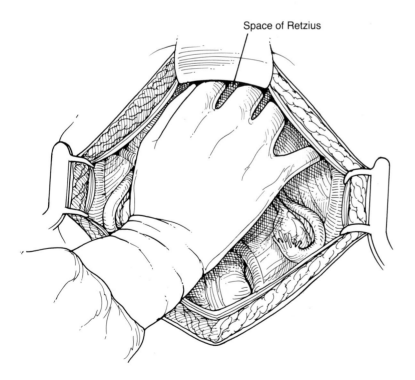

Figure 5-2. A midline, Cherney, or Maylard incision is made to the level of the peritoneum. Once the transversalis fascia has been incised laterally, the space of Retzius is developed. The weight of the operator's hand in the midline separates the bladder from the overlying symphysis. Once the bladder is mobilized in the central portion, blunt dissection with the operator's hand or a sponge stick can further develop the paravesical space, and the peritoneum can easily be dissected from the lateral pelvic sidewalls.

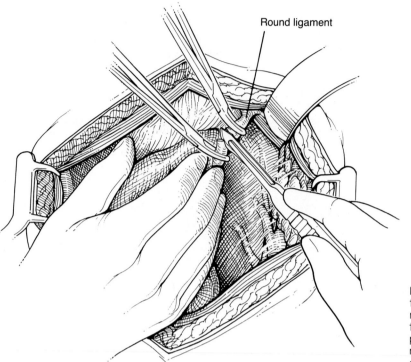

Round ligament

Figure 5-3. Sectioning the round ligament extraperitoneally at its exit through the inguinal ring will further develop the lateral spaces. At this point, the finger of the operator can be placed anterior to the external iliac vessels to mobilize tissue cephalad to the level of the common iliac vessels.

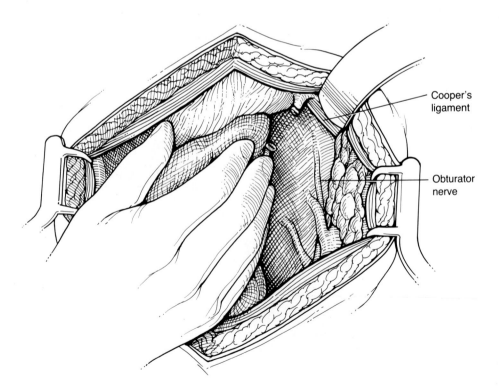

Cooper's ligament

Obturator nerve

Figure 5-4. The pelvic space is completely exposed. The obturator nerve is noted deep in the pelvis. Cooper's ligament should also be identified. Venous oozing may occur at the site of attachment of the peritoneum to Cooper's ligament and can be controlled with cautery.

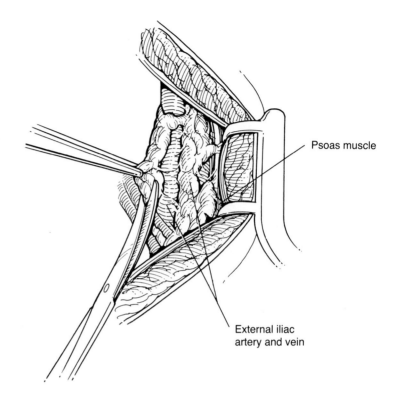

Psoas muscle

External iliac
artery and vein

Figure 5–5. Starting at the bifurcation of the common iliac vessels, the loose areolar tissue over the vein is excised from cephalad to caudad. Clips should be used at the bifurcation of the common iliac to avoid troublesome bleeding.

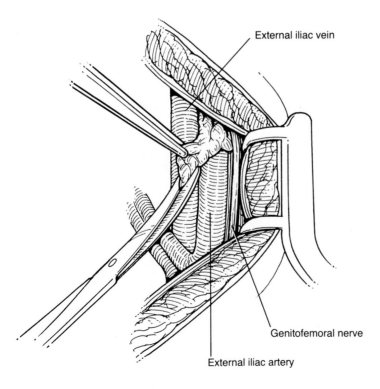

External iliac vein

Genitofemoral nerve

External iliac artery

Figure 5–6. The fibroareolar tissue over the external iliac artery is mobilized in a similar fashion from cephalad to caudad. The genitofemoral nerve, seen on the lateral border of the external iliac artery, should be identified prior to excising lymphatic tissue. Clips or a tie should be used on the cephalad bundle, at the level of the common iliac bifurcation.

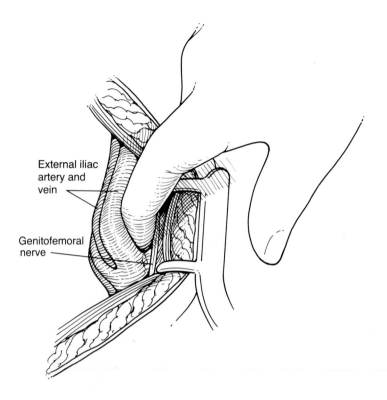

External iliac
artery and
vein

Genitofemoral
nerve

Figure 5–7. Once the external iliac vessels have been cleared of lymphatic tissue, the finger of the operator is passed lateral to these vessels in order to free tissue in the obturator space. The finger should be inserted gently.

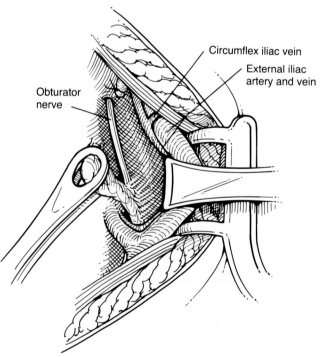

Circumflex iliac vein

External iliac
artery and vein

Obturator
nerve

Figure 5–8. A vein retractor is used to retract the external iliac veins anterior and lateral to expose the obturator space. Lymphatic tissue is gently teased from the psoas muscle. The entire lymphatic bundle is clamped, sectioned at its caudal end, and ligated at the pelvic sidewall. With the use of the Singley forceps, the lymphatic bundle is bluntly dissected from the obturator nerve and mobilized superiorly. Often, the obturator vein and artery must be sacrificed to obtain access to tissue posterior and lateral to the nerve. Once the tissue is mobilized superiorly, all areolar tissue is cleaned off the hypogastric vessels to the level of the bifurcation of the common iliac artery. The large tissue bundle is clamped and removed en bloc. A tie or suture may be used.

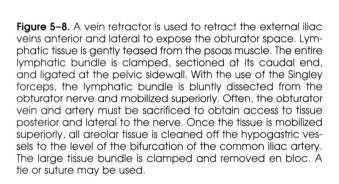

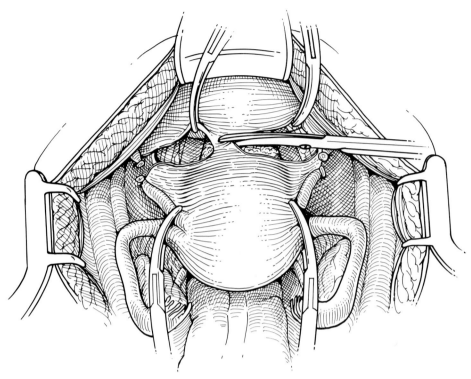

Figure 5–9. The hysterectomy. The peritoneum of the avascular layer of the anterior broad ligament is incised bilaterally. The paravesical space is further developed bilaterally. This may be done by gently teasing away the areolar tissue with the finger of the operator, pushing the tissue medially. The peritoneum between the spaces is sectioned.

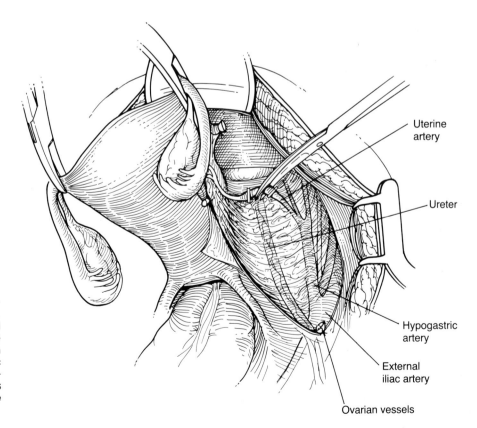

Figure 5–10. The uterine artery is transected as it crosses over the ureter. Vascular clips may be used instead of clamps. The uterine vein may be separately clamped or clipped. In this drawing, the infundibulopelvic ligament has been previously sectioned and the lateral spaces opened. In the young patient, the ovaries may be preserved.

Uterine artery

Ureter

Hypogastric artery

External iliac artery

Ovarian vessels

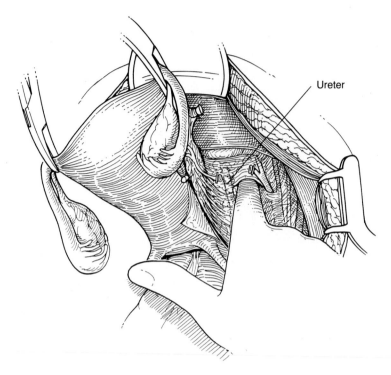

Ureter

Figure 5–11. Once the uterine artery is ligated, the pararectal space is developed by the finger of the operator. The rectum is pushed medially in this avascular space. Care must be taken to avoid injury to the posteriorly lying hypogastric vein. These steps are repeated on the opposite side.

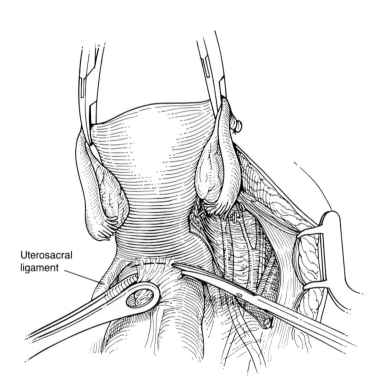

Uterosacral ligament

Figure 5–12. The rectovaginal space is then developed. The rectosigmoid is grasped loosely with ring forceps and an incision is made between the uterosacral ligaments. With blunt and sharp dissection, the rectum can be easily separated from the posterior vagina.

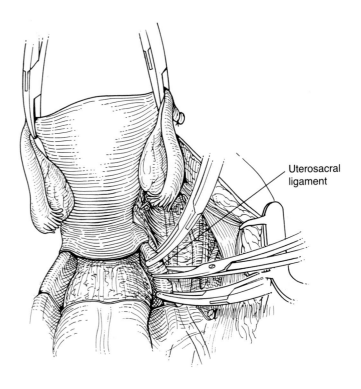

Uterosacral
ligament

Figure 5–13. With all spaces developed, the uterosacral ligaments are clamped halfway from the uterus to their sacral attachments. The uterus must be kept on constant traction by the assistant so that the surgeon can clearly visualize the uterosacral ligaments. Suturing the medial and cephalad clamp initially will allow better exposure for the eventual suture ligation to the remaining tissue bundle. In this drawing, the pararectal space is noted laterally, and the rectovaginal space is medial to the uterosacral ligament. By removing the posterior attachments earlier in the operation, the surgeon makes the uterus more mobile, and removing the ureter from its tunnel is more easily accomplished.

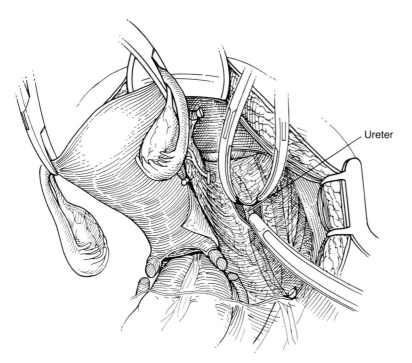

Ureter

Figure 5–14. The ureter is unroofed from the tunnel of tissue that contains uterine vessels and its branches by the use of a scoop developed by Uchida. This scoop, with grooves on both sides, is inserted into the triangulated tissue making up the anterior portion of the tunnel.

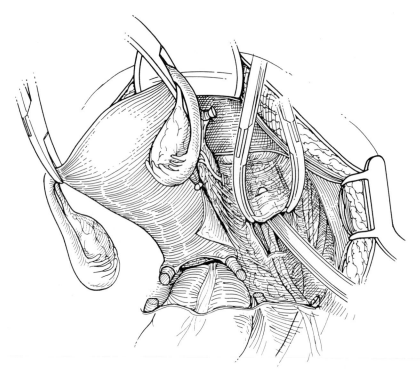

Figure 5–15. The scoop is inserted into the tunnel. The ureter is located posterior to the scoop. The groove in the posterior portion of the scoop allows the ureter to be protected when this maneuver is performed. The scoop is passed cephalad and lateral to medial. Care must be taken to avoid inserting the scoop into the bladder.

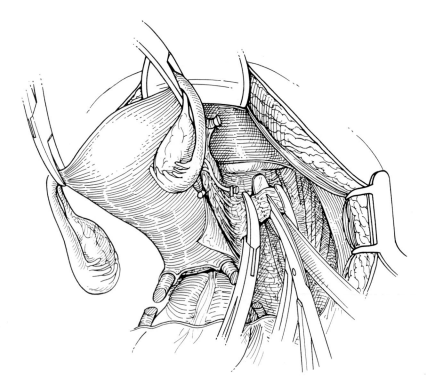

Figure 5–16. The anterior vesico-uterine ligament is incised between two Moynihan clamps. The lateral forceps can be turned to the side to visualize the medial and posterior attachments. With the modified radical hysterectomy, these attachments should be left intact.

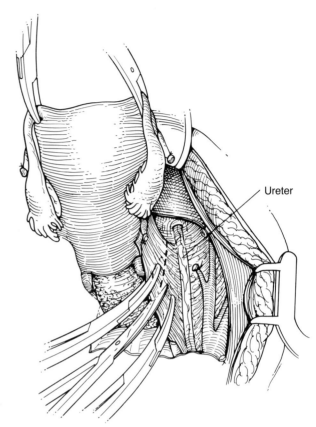

Figure 5-17. With the ureter unroofed but still attached to the posterior peritoneum, the cardinal ligament is transected halfway from its origin from the uterus and its insertion on the lateral pelvic sidewall. Note the ureters rolled laterally and posteriorly, far removed from the inserted clamps. Several bites may be needed to transect the cardinal ligament.

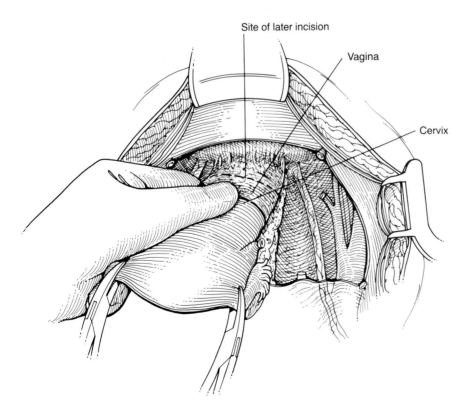

Figure 5-18. The uterus is pulled to the opposite side and the cervix is palpated. Approximately the upper third of the vagina should be included in the specimen. Note that the ureter is still attached posteriorly to the peritoneum. This maneuver allows one to judge adequate placement of clamps on the vagina. Often, a tag suture can be used prior to placing the clamp.

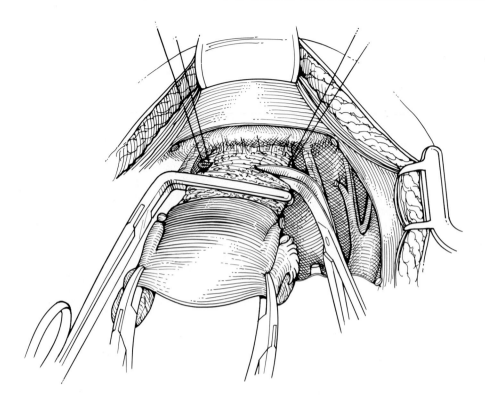

Figure 5-19. A large right-angle clamp is placed to include the upper third of the vagina. Stay sutures may be used for the lateral vaginal angles. The right-angled Jorgenson scissors are used to section the vagina below the clamp. The vagina may be closed with figure-of-eight sutures or a running suture. Retroperitoneal drains are placed. We only suture the peritoneum over the bladder to the peritoneum over the rectum, but otherwise do not reperitonealize.

REFERENCES

1. DiSaia PJ: The case against the surgical concept of en bloc dissection for certain malignancies of the reproductive tract. Cancer 60:2025–2034, 1987.
2. Downey GO, Potish PA, Adcock LL, et al: Pretreatment surgical staging in cervical carcinoma: Therapeutic efficacy of pelvic lymph node dissection. Obstet Gynecol 160:1055–1061, 1989.
3. Meigs JV: Carcinoma of the cervix—The Wertheim operation. Surg Gynecol Obstet 78:195, 1944.
4. Photopulos GJ, Zwagg RV: Class II radical hysterectomy shows less morbidity and good efficacy compared to class III. Gynecol Oncol 40:21–24, 1991.
5. Piver MS, Rutledge F, Smith JP: Five classes of extended hysterectomy for women with cervical cancer. Obstet Gynecol 44:265–272, 1974.
6. Uchida H: Radical operation for cancer of the cervix (on the basis of 3,240 operations). Proceedings of Tenth World Congress of Gynecology and Obstetrics, San Francisco, 1982.
7. Wertheim E: The extended abdominal operation for carcinoma uteri. Am J Obstet Gynecol 69:33, 1955.

6

Radical Hysterectomy with Pelvic Lymph Node Dissection

The operation is designed to remove the uterus with or without the adnexa, various lengths of vaginal canal (most often the upper third), the entire parametrium, uterosacral ligaments, vesicouterine ligaments, pelvic nodes, lower common and external iliac nodes, and obturator and hypogastric nodes. Parametrial and ureteral nodes are removed along with the cardinal ligament and are not in themselves part of the node dissection per se. The procedure, as here depicted, is employed in patients with stages I-B and II-A cancer of the cervix.

Pathophysiologic changes revolve mainly around the urinary tract as a result of ureteral and bladder dissection. Most patients with class III radical hysterectomies will develop a neurogenic bladder soon after the surgery that may require close attention for several weeks. Although the majority of the patients recover, some continue to have a neurogenic hypotonic bladder, whereas others develop bladder instability. Patients undergoing radical hysterectomy for cancer of the cervix need to have their urinary system monitored yearly for the first 2 years and every 3 to 5 years thereafter. Such monitoring will provide information regarding complications of surgery as well as monitor the disease itself.

Prior to surgery, the patient is evaluated with pertinent diagnostic tests, e.g., intravenous pyelography (IVP), barium enema, cystoscopy, proctoscopy, laboratory tests to indicate the nutritional status, and hepatic and urinary function tests. The gastrointestinal (GI) tract, as for any pelvic oncologic procedure, is prepared with any of the several bowel preparation protocols available. The night prior to surgery, a triple-lumen catheter is inserted into a central vein for fluid and blood administration as well as for monitoring central venous pressure.

POTENTIAL PROBLEM AREAS

These steps in the operation offer potential risks: (1) vessel injury during dissection of the pelvic wall may occur while performing lymph node dissection, because of frequent anatomic variation of the branches of the hypogastric vessels; (2) if the blood supply to the distal ureter is not preserved, or if the dissection is carried too close to the ureter, strictures and fistulas may develop; and (3) too vigorous dissection of the bladder base may weaken its wall, and fistula formation may result.

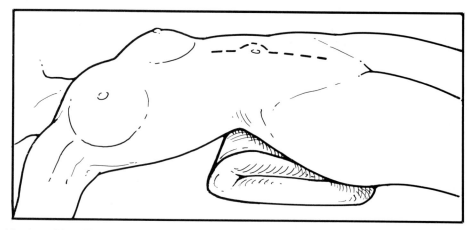

Figure 6–1. Patient is placed in a "jack-knife" position to improve visualization of pelvic contents. Two or three rolled sheets are placed underneath the hips, the table is tilted to a 30-degree Trendelenburg position with the foot of the table lowered. The abdomen is opened through a midline incision extended to the left and above the umbilicus. The abdomen is explored in a systematic fashion. A detailed description can be found in Chapter 10, Total Pelvic Exenteration.

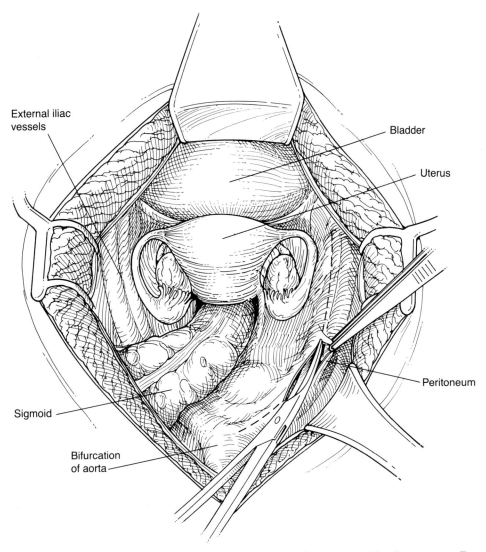

External iliac
vessels

Bladder

Uterus

Peritoneum

Sigmoid

Bifurcation
of aorta

Figure 6–2. After obtaining pelvic washings for cytologic evaluation, the peritoneum overlying the common iliac vessels is opened. The incision is extended cephalad to the bifurcation of the aorta and distally to the inguinal ligaments.

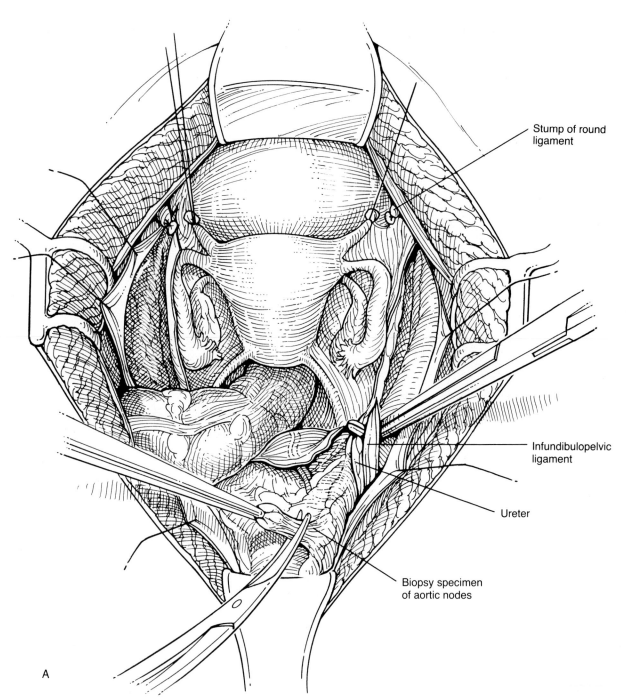

Stump of round
ligament

Infundibulopelvic
ligament

Ureter

Biopsy specimen
of aortic nodes

A

Figure 6–3. *A,* Biopsies of aortic and caval nodes are obtained and submitted for frozen section. If pathologic evaluation reveals metastatic disease, the operation is abandoned. The round ligament is cut and ligated close to the pelvic wall. The infundibulo-pelvic ligament is isolated and the ovarian vessels are ligated and cut. *B,* Exposure of the retroperitoneal area with the ureter attached to the medial leaf of the broad ligament.

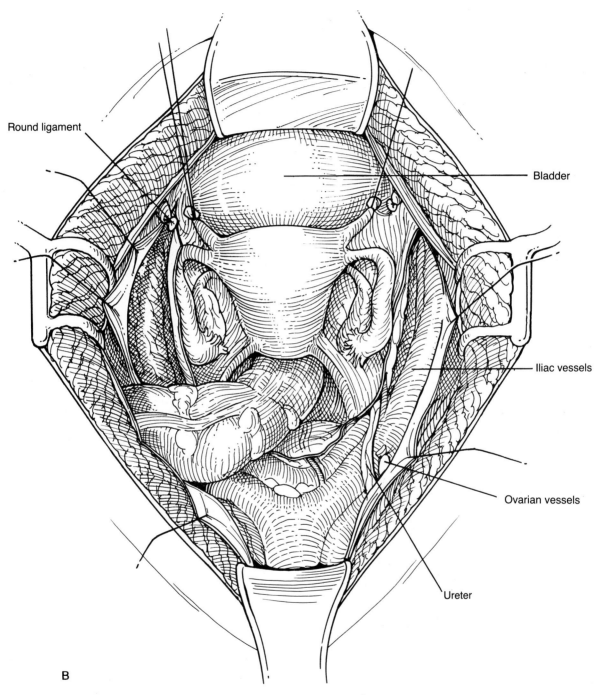

Round ligament

Bladder

Iliac vessels

Ovarian vessels

Ureter

B

Figure 6–3 *See legend on opposite page.*

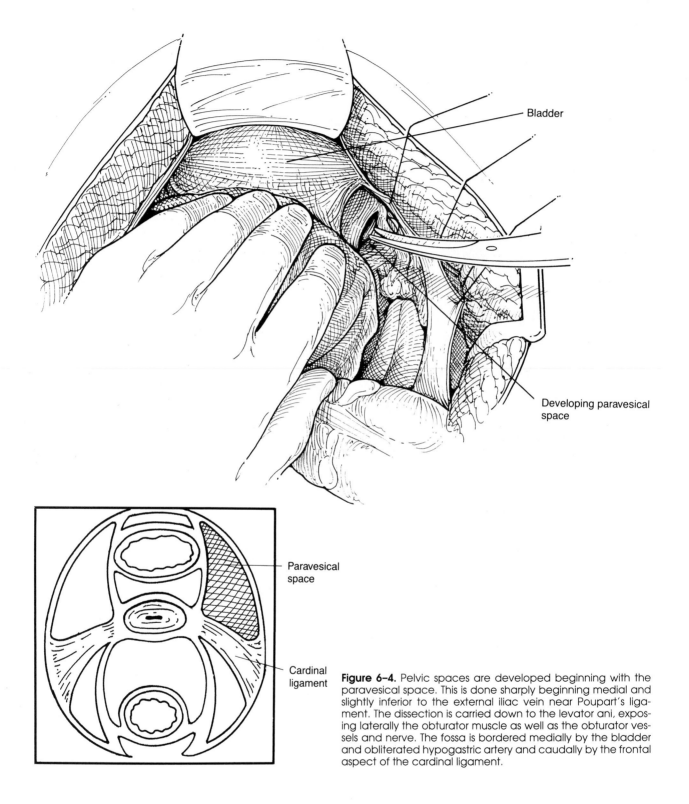

Bladder

Developing paravesical
space

Paravesical
space

Cardinal
ligament

Figure 6–4. Pelvic spaces are developed beginning with the paravesical space. This is done sharply beginning medial and slightly inferior to the external iliac vein near Poupart's ligament. The dissection is carried down to the levator ani, exposing laterally the obturator muscle as well as the obturator vessels and nerve. The fossa is bordered medially by the bladder and obliterated hypogastric artery and caudally by the frontal aspect of the cardinal ligament.

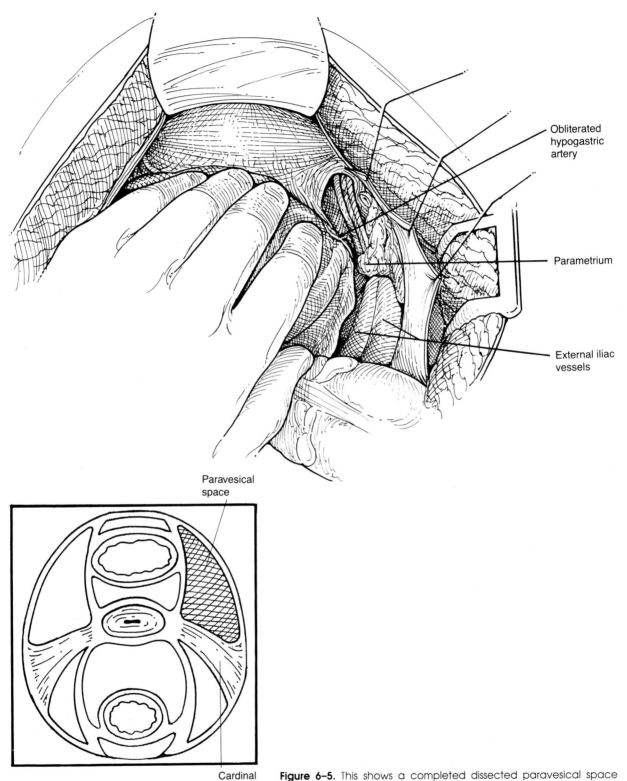

Obliterated
hypogastric
artery

Parametrium

External iliac
vessels

Paravesical
space

Cardinal
ligament

Figure 6–5. This shows a completed dissected paravesical space with the anatomical structures as indicated in the previous figure.

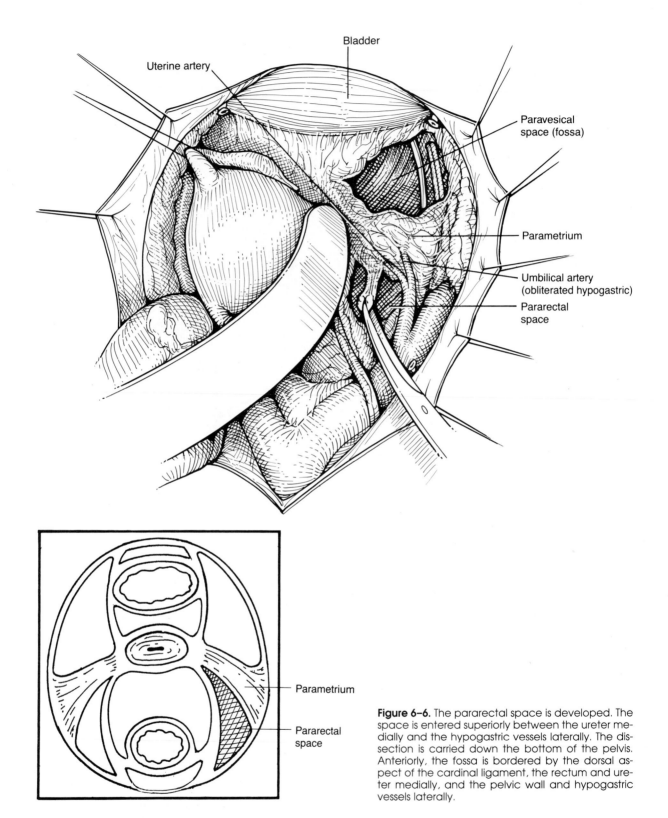

Bladder

Uterine artery

Paravesical space (fossa)

Parametrium

Umbilical artery (obliterated hypogastric)

Pararectal space

Parametrium

Pararectal space

Figure 6-6. The pararectal space is developed. The space is entered superiorly between the ureter medially and the hypogastric vessels laterally. The dissection is carried down the bottom of the pelvis. Anteriorly, the fossa is bordered by the dorsal aspect of the cardinal ligament, the rectum and ureter medially, and the pelvic wall and hypogastric vessels laterally.

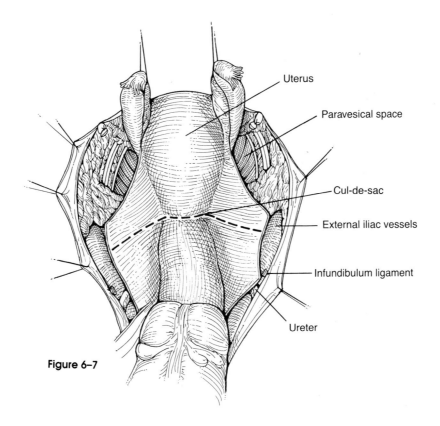

Uterus

Paravesical space

Cul-de-sac

External iliac vessels

Infundibulum ligament

Ureter

Figure 6–7

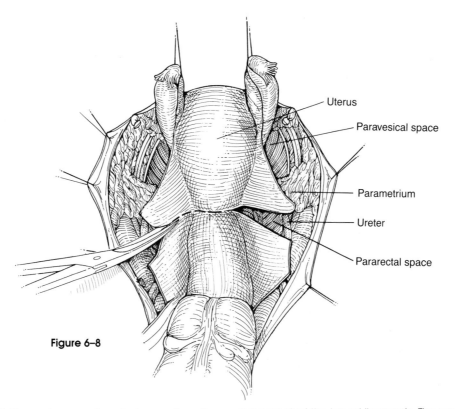

Uterus

Paravesical space

Parametrium

Ureter

Pararectal space

Figure 6–8

Figures 6–7 and 6–8. The ureters are dissected away from the medial aspect of the broad ligaments. The peritoneum between the ureters across the cul-de-sac is incised in preparation for development of the rectovaginal space.

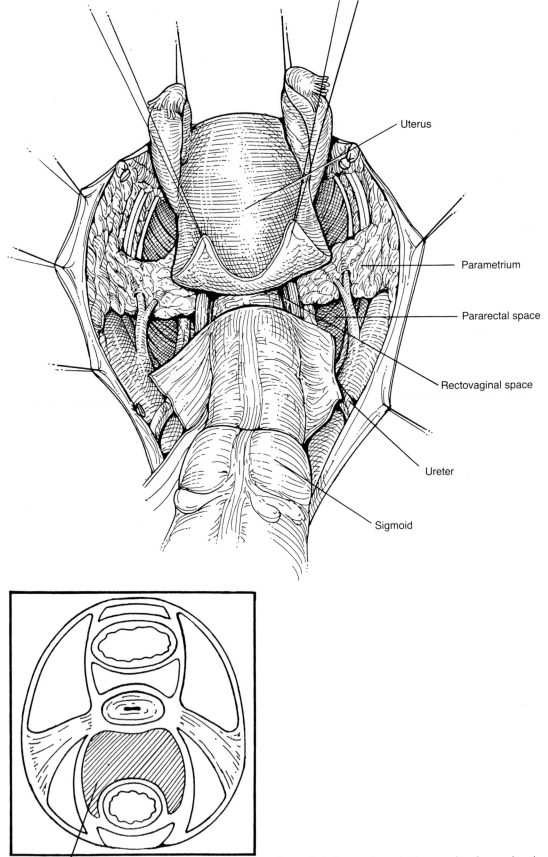

Uterus

Parametrium

Pararectal space

Rectovaginal space

Ureter

Sigmoid

Rectovaginal space

Figure 6-9. The rectovaginal space has been developed, freeing the uterus from its posterior visceral attachments.

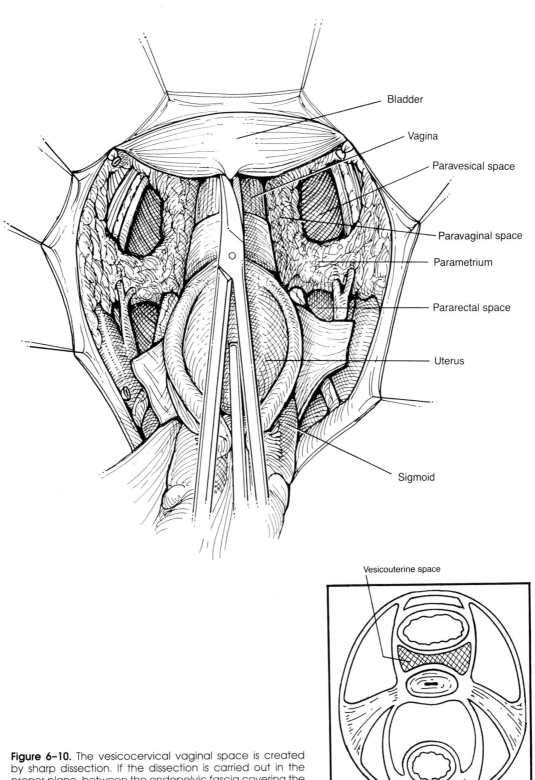

Bladder

Vagina

Paravesical space

Paravaginal space

Parametrium

Pararectal space

Uterus

Sigmoid

Vesicouterine space

Figure 6-10. The vesicocervical vaginal space is created by sharp dissection. If the dissection is carried out in the proper plane, between the endopelvic fascia covering the cervix and vagina on one side and the bladder on the opposite side, it is usually bloodless and simple.

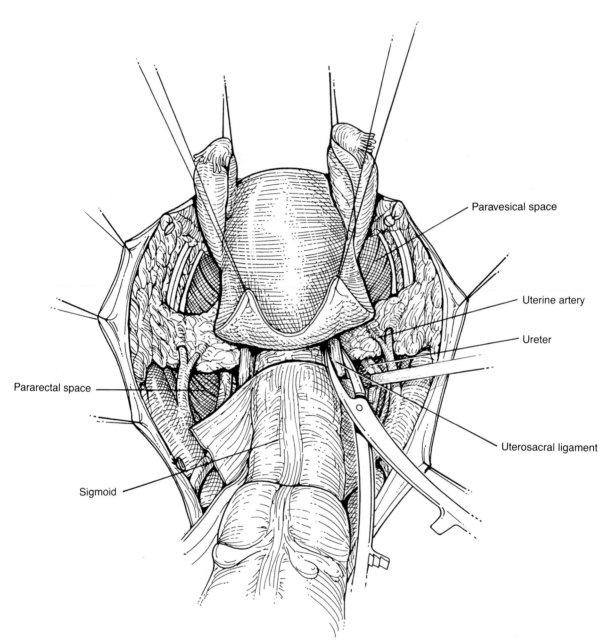

Paravesical space

Uterine artery

Ureter

Uterosacral ligament

Pararectal space

Sigmoid

Figure 6–11. The uterosacral ligaments are clamped close to their insertion on the pelvis posteriorly.

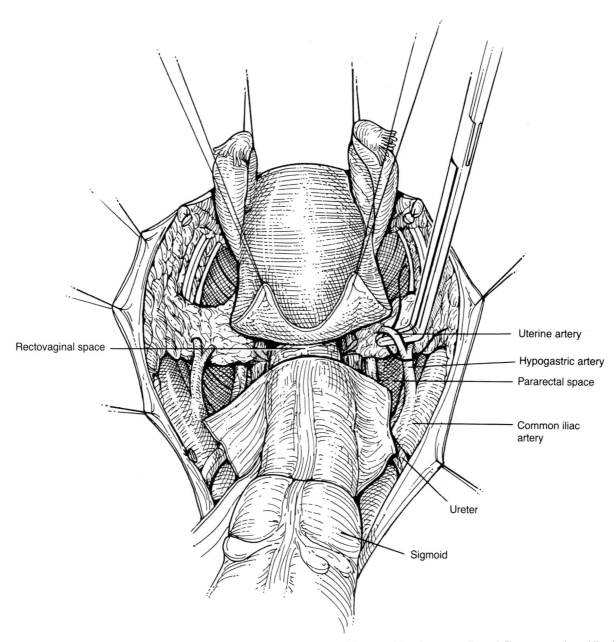

Rectovaginal space

Uterine artery

Hypogastric artery

Pararectal space

Common iliac artery

Ureter

Sigmoid

Figure 6–12. The uterine vessels are exposed easily once the uterosacral ligament has been sectioned. They are cut and ligated close to their origin in the hypogastric vessels.

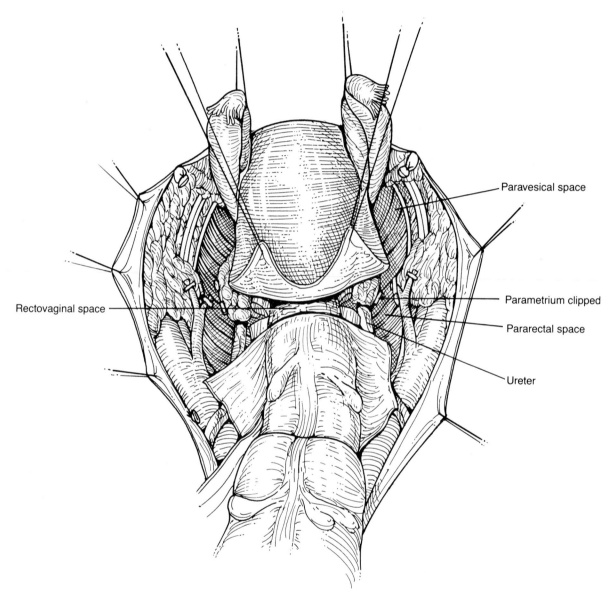

Rectovaginal space

Paravesical space

Parametrium clipped

Pararectal space

Ureter

Figure 6–13. The cardinal ligament is now either serially clamped, cut, and ligated to the pelvic floor, or, alternatively, the ligament is dissected out and the parametrial vessels are individually ligated or clipped and cut.

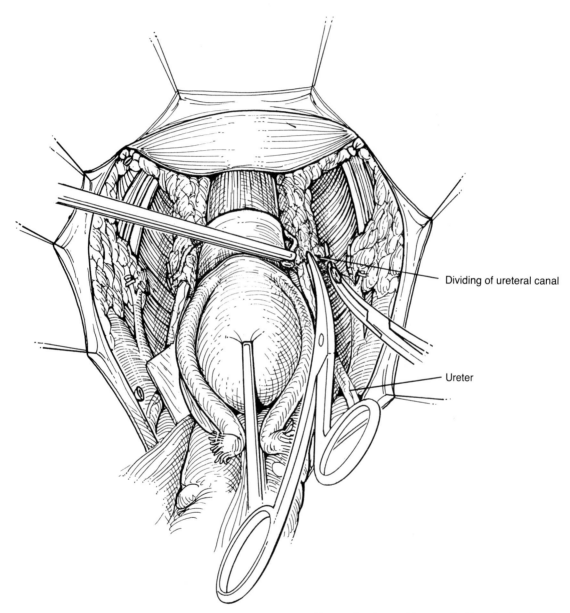

Dividing of ureteral canal

Ureter

Figure 6–14. Dissection of the ureter from the parametrium is begun. The ureteral canal is unroofed by placing traction on the medial stump of the uterine vessels.

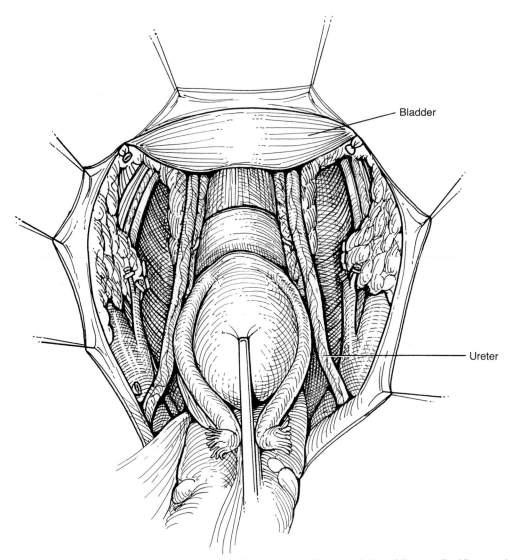

Bladder

Ureter

Figure 6–15. Paravesical space and pararectal space united after sectioning the remainder of the cardinal ligaments. The ureters can be seen in their trajectory from the infundibulopelvic ligament down to the bladder.

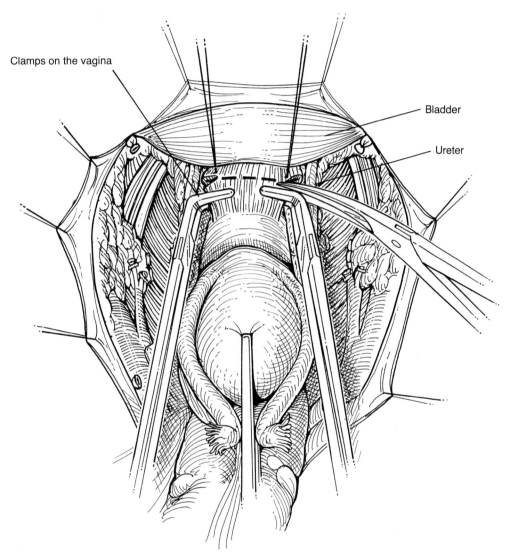

Clamps on the vagina

Bladder

Ureter

Figure 6–16. Right-angle clamps are applied to the vagina in preparation for removal of the specimen.

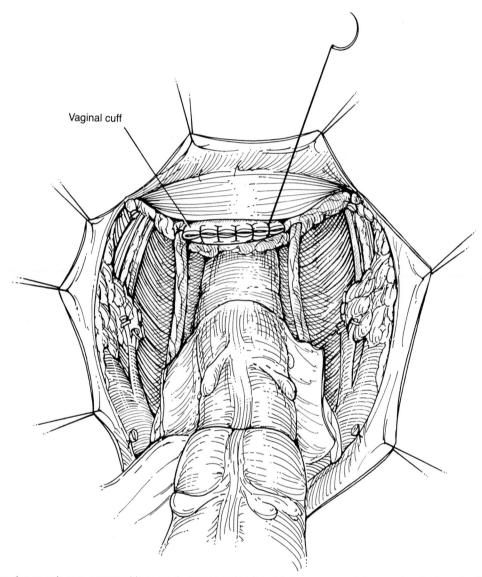

Vaginal cuff

Figure 6–17. The uterus, adnexa, parametrium, and upper vagina have been removed; the vagina is closed with 2-0 absorbable polyglycolic acid sutures.

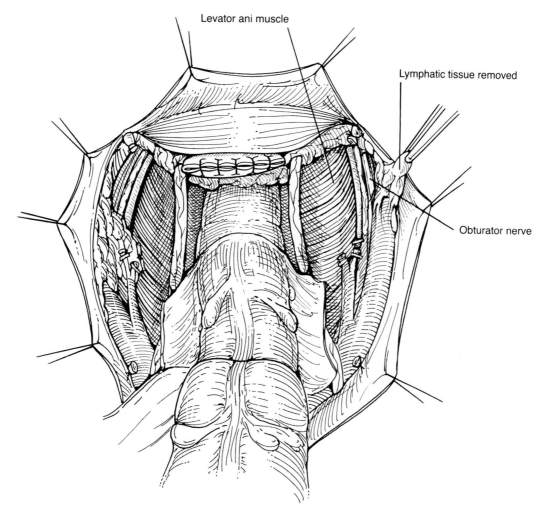

Levator ani muscle

Lymphatic tissue removed

Obturator nerve

Figure 6–18. Beginning of lymphadenectomy, which is performed from the common iliac vessels down to the inguinal ligaments. Prior removal of the specimen makes this part of the operation simpler; alternatively, it can be done at the beginning of the procedure prior to resecting the uterus and parametrium.

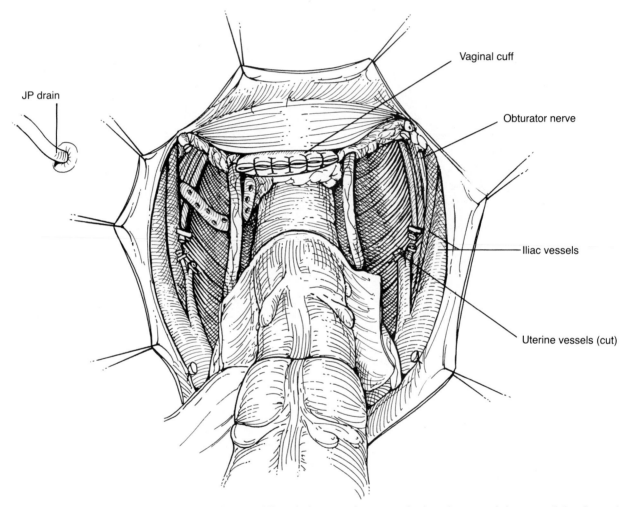

JP drain

Vaginal cuff

Obturator nerve

Iliac vessels

Uterine vessels (cut)

Figure 6–19. Completed operation with the stumps of the uterine vessels, paravesical and pararectal spaces (joined), vaginal vault closed, dissection of the lower rectosigmoid, and lymphadenectomy.

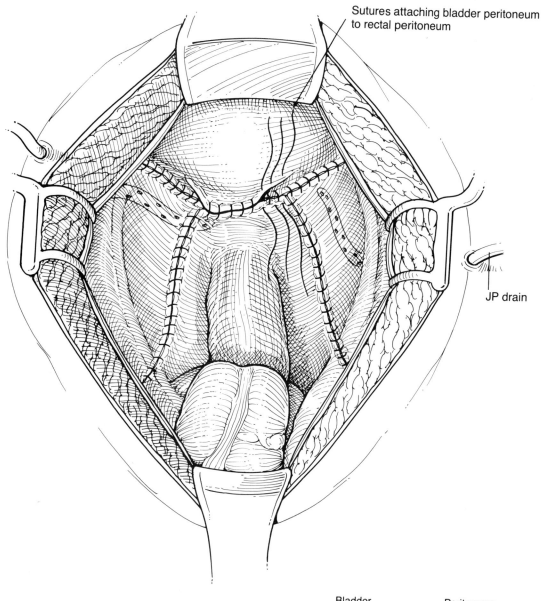

Sutures attaching bladder peritoneum to rectal peritoneum

JP drain

Bladder

Peritoneum

Rectum

Figure 6–20. Two approaches can be taken to the denuded pelvis. The first is to place Jackson-Pratt drains in the most dependent portion of the pelvis and close the abdomen with continuous massive type of closure. Alternatively, the pelvic perito-neum is closed as depicted on the illustration. Drains are left in the retroperitoneal space. Early in our experience, we created a pocket of perito-neum in hopes of enlarging the shortened vaginal canal. In recent years, we have eliminated this step and have not seen any major differences postop-eratively.

BIBLIOGRAPHY

Liu W, Meigs JW: Radical hysterectomy and pelvic lymphadenectomy. Am J Obstet Gynecol 69:1, 1955.

Meigs JV (ed): Surgical Treatment of Cancer of Cervix. Grune and Stratton, New York, 1954, pp 149–196.

Parsons L, Ulfelder H: An Atlas of Pelvic Operations. WB Saunders Co, Philadelphia, 1968, pp 324–349.

Piver MS, Rutledge FN, Smith PJ: Five classes of extended hysterectomy of women with cervical cancer. Obstet Gynecol 44:265, 1974.

Wheeless C: Atlas of Pelvic Surgery. Lea and Febiger, Philadelphia, 1981, pp 360–363.

7

Surgery for Advanced Ovarian Cancer

Mark J. Messing, M.D.

The surgical management of ovarian cancer consists of the removal of the diseased ovary or ovaries and debulking of metastatic cancer implants. Several studies have demonstrated that maximal surgical excision results in improved survival when combined with chemotherapy.[5–10] The optimal extent of surgical excision is still under debate regarding the smallest acceptable residual tumor nodule. Debulking individual tumor nodules to less than 2 cm is a generally accepted goal in most patients. Success with so-called optimal debulking has been achieved in 28 to 72 per cent of published series.[2, 3, 5]

The approach to advanced ovarian cancer takes advantage of the knowledge that ovarian cancer tends to be a peritoneal surface disease. Even in the face of bulky pelvic and omental disease, a dissection plane can often be created between the malignant process and viscera or peritoneum. Following surgical debulking of large disease, additional measures can be undertaken utilizing new technology such as ultrasonic destruction of implants (CUSA) or electrical destruction with the argon beam coagulator (ABC).

Surgical debulking of advanced ovarian cancer can be undertaken only through a generous midline incision. An initial thorough exploration of the peritoneal cavity will define the extent of surface disease and involvement of intra-abdominal structures. Removing large-volume omental disease is often of significant palliative benefit in controlling ascites and improving symptoms related to abdominal distention. Quality of life has been shown to be improved in patients who undergo aggressive debulking surgery.[1] Removal or partial resection of other intra-abdominal organs should be performed only in those cases where specific palliation (bowel obstruction) or optimal tumor debulking will result. Intestinal surgery has been reported in 13 to 20 per cent of aggressively approached cases.[2, 5] Splenectomy is rarely required, but has been performed to achieve optimal debulking. Trauma to the spleen during omentectomy may occur from vigorous traction and is probably the most frequent indication for removal.[6] In general, removal of peritoneal implants larger than 2 cm should be performed. Aggressive attempts to remove nodules smaller than 1 cm or extensive plaque disease can add considerable time to the procedure with unclear associated benefit.

The key to approaching extensive pelvic disease involves knowledge of the retroperitoneal anatomy and the free spaces between the pelvic structures. A retroperitoneal dissection will allow the surgeon to place vital structures such as the ureter and the ovarian and pelvic vessels under direct visualization in order to avoid injury. Dissection from the lateral pelvis to the midline allows for early control of the blood supply and mobilizes the pelvic structures so that clamps can be applied more easily and safely. En-bloc dissection of the pelvic organs is not required. The early removal of bulky ovarian disease prior to hysterectomy is reasonable and facilitates exposure. Sigmoid disease can often be debulked without resorting to bowel resection, once the large primary ovarian disease is resected.

If significant sigmoid disease remains as the main area of bulky residual, resection and primary reanastomosis can be performed. Occasionally, the pelvic structures are so "frozen" that a dissection between sigmoid and uterus cannot be attempted from cephalad to caudad. The technique of reverse hysterectomy can often identify the rectovaginal plane and allow for separation of the uterus from the sigmoid. Adequate intestinal preparation prior to surgery in anticipation of a possible sigmoid resection will ease any concerns should the bowel be entered. Preoperative barium enema or sigmoidoscopy will rule out any intrinsic disease that might call for sigmoid resection.

Bladder involvement is rarely a problem in advanced ovarian cancer. Dense involvement of the vesicouterine peritoneum with tumor can often be debulked along with excision of the anterior pelvic peritoneum. This will then allow access to the plane between bladder and uterus. A lateral approach from the paravesical space can help identify the ideal dissection plane and avoid the hazards of dissecting through a thickened, redundant peritoneum.

POTENTIAL COMPLICATIONS

The main difficulties experienced in removing extensive pelvic cancer are blood loss and lack of exposure. Identification of the retroperitoneal anatomy early in the dissection is key. The ovarian vessels should be ligated early once the ureter is visualized and safely retracted. Separation of the ureter from its peritoneal attachments, similar to a radical hysterectomy, will allow a safer dissection if the adnexa are adherent to the posterior peritoneum. Dissection of the ureter from its parametrial course is usually not necessary. Adequate preoperative intestinal preparation is essential to decompress the bowel and prevent spillage of fecal material in the event of an enterotomy. In such cases, primary repair of an enterotomy is appropriate.

PATHOPHYSIOLOGIC CHANGES

The ultimate goal of an aggressive surgical approach to advanced ovarian cancer is maximal resection of all visible tumor. Blood and tissue fluid loss from large areas of denuded pelvic peritoneum is difficult to quantitate but can continue for days after surgery. Large volumes of ascites may be removed at the initial exploration. The operative team needs to be continuously aware of these insensible fluid losses and to closely monitor the patient's vital signs and urine output. Central venous monitoring may assist in the appropriate replacement of fluid volume. Those patients who had significant ascites prior to surgery will tend to reaccumulate this fluid to some degree after surgery. The early administra-

tion of chemotherapy may help to control ascites reaccumulation.

Intestinal ileus may persist for several days after surgery depending on the extent of intraperitoneal disease. Patients who present with significant malnutrition or those who may be expected to have a prolonged recovery of over 1 week should be considered for nutritional supplementation. Intravenous hyperalimentation or enteral feeding by intraoperative placement of a feeding jejunostomy or gastrostomy may be appropriate in these selected cases.

PART I. RADICAL DEBULKING FOR OVARIAN CANCER

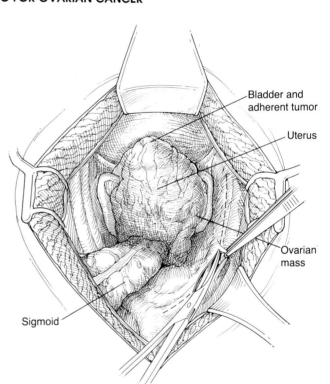

Figure 7-1. The small intestine, sigmoid, and cecum have been packed into the upper abdomen and the pelvis is exposed. A large adherent pelvic mass involving the ovaries, sigmoid colon, and anterior and posterior peritoneal surfaces is depicted. Dissection begins by entering the posterior retroperitoneum lateral to the external iliac vessels.

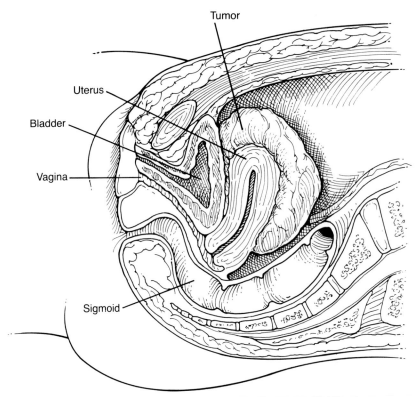

Figure 7–2. A lateral view of the pelvis depicts the extent of the ovarian mass, which is adherent to the uterus and to the anterior and posterior cul-de-sac.

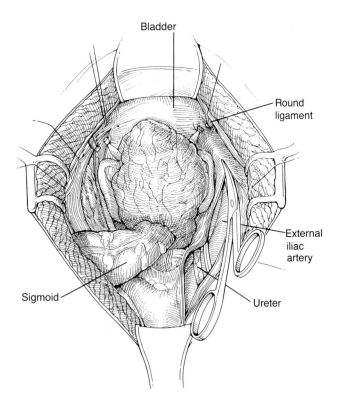

Figure 7–3. After opening the posteror peritoneum, the surgeon identifies the iliac vessels. The ovarian vessels and ureter cross at the bifurcation of the internal and external iliac vessels. The round ligament is divided.

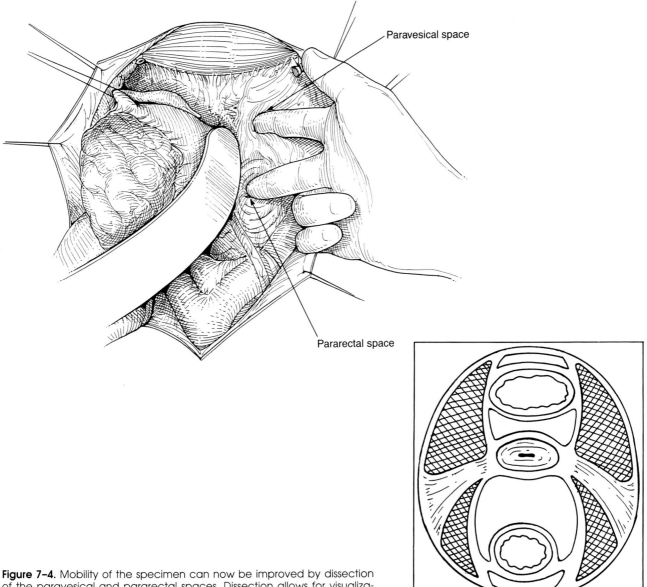

Paravesical space

Pararectal space

Figure 7–4. Mobility of the specimen can now be improved by dissection of the paravesical and pararectal spaces. Dissection allows for visualization of the ureter into the pelvis as well as the pelvic vessels.

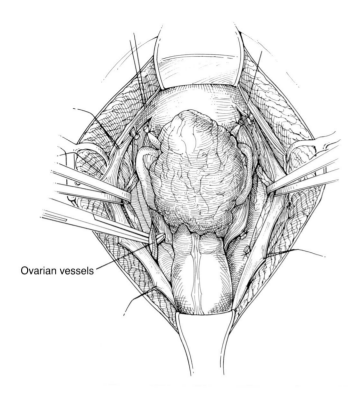

Ovarian vessels

Figure 7–5. The ovarian vessels are skeletonized and divided at the pelvic brim. Early control of these vessels will help reduce blood loss during the later dissection. The ureter can be mobilized off the medial leaf of the broad ligament and retracted laterally on a Penrose drain.

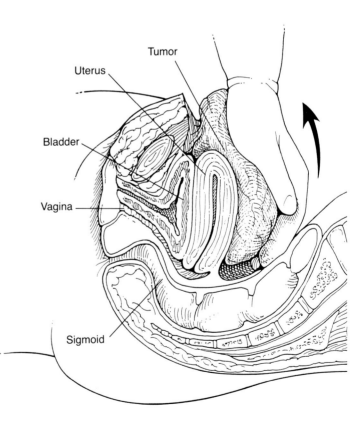

Tumor

Uterus

Bladder

Vagina

Sigmoid

Figure 7–6. Further mobilization of the ovaries can be obtained by blunt dissection off of the rectosigmoid. If the adherence of the mass to the sigmoid is suggestive of invasion, an approach by the ''reverse'' hysterectomy method is employed (see Figures 7–22 through 7–30).

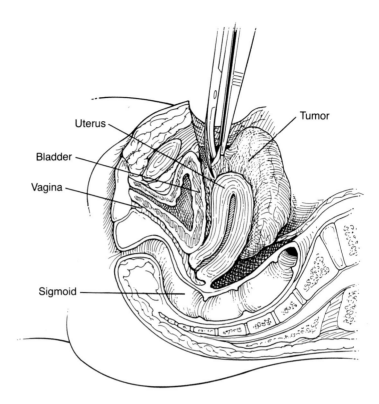

Figure 7-7. Opening the peritoneum over the bladder should start well above the tumor edge. Because the typical ovarian cancer is a surface disease, a plane can usually be found to mobilize the peritoneal disease off of the bladder. The vesicocervical plane is usually unaffected by this disease.

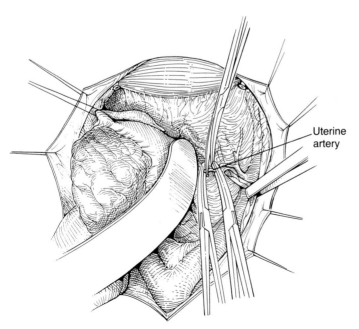

Figure 7-8. The uterine artery is divided medial to the ureter if possible. Occasionally the volume of disease is such that division lateral to the ureter is required and the medial half of the vessel must be mobilized off of the ureter.

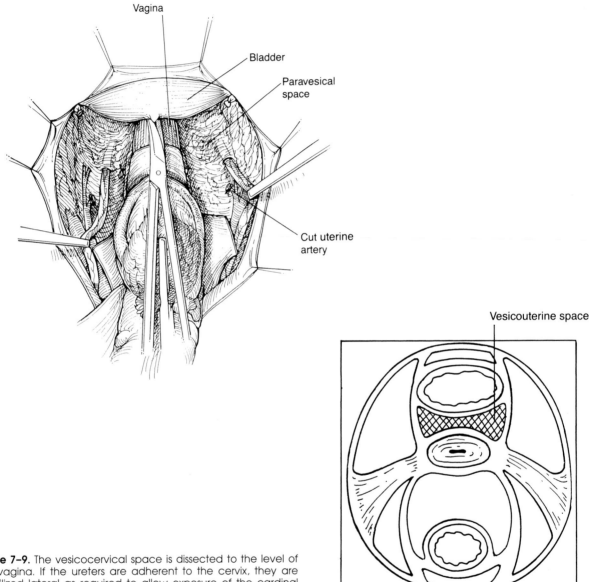

Figure 7–9. The vesicocervical space is dissected to the level of the vagina. If the ureters are adherent to the cervix, they are mobilized lateral as required to allow exposure of the cardinal and uterosacral ligaments.

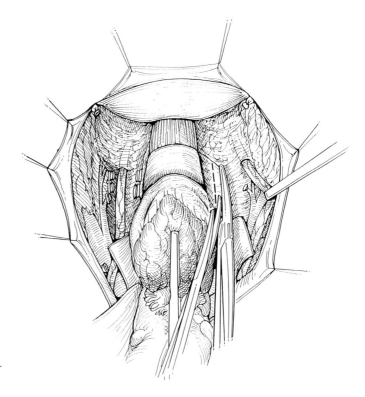

Figure 7-10. The ureters are retracted laterally as the cardinal ligaments and uterosacral ligaments are divided.

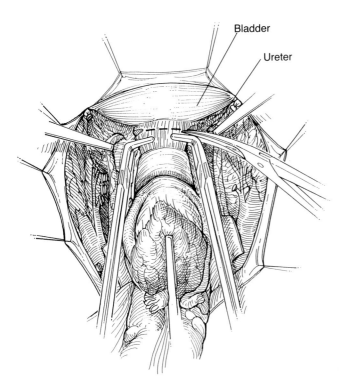

Bladder

Ureter

Figure 7-11. The vaginal angles are clamped and the specimen is separated from the vagina.

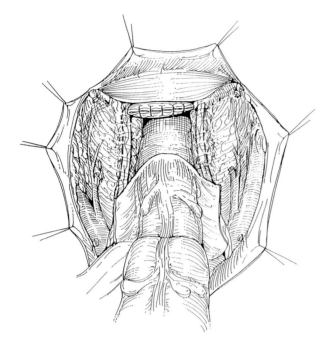

Figure 7-12. The vaginal mucosa is closed with interrupted sutures.

PART II. OMENTECTOMY AND GASTROSTOMY

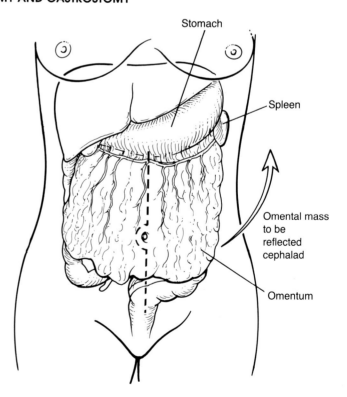

Stomach

Spleen

Omental mass to be reflected cephalad

Omentum

Figure 7-13. An extended midline incision is required to expose the transverse colon and stomach to facilitate the dissection of the omentum. Reflecting the omentum cephalad exposes the reflection of the omentum where it joins the transverse colon. Even with an omentum extensively involved with tumor, this plane can be identified and can allow entry into the lesser sac.

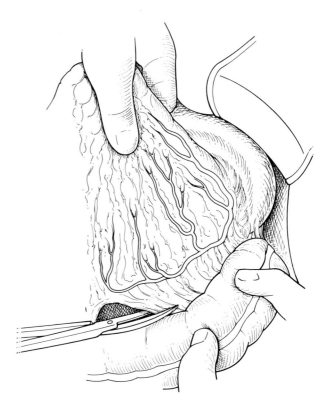

Figure 7–14. Separation of the omentum off the transverse colon along its undersurface can be accomplished in an avascular plane. After entering the lesser sac, the omentum can be extensively mobilized and its attachments to the stomach better defined. Care should be taken to avoid dissection into the mesentery of the transverse colon in more difficult cases.

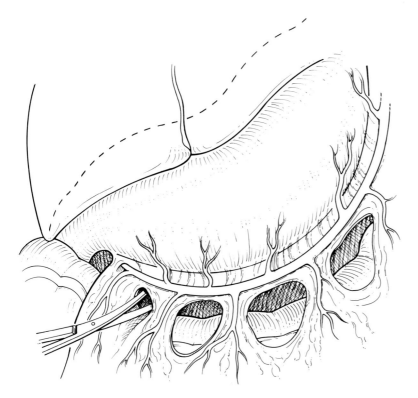

Figure 7–15. Once the omentum has been satisfactorily mobilized, the superior extent of the dissection can be defined. Extensive debulking of tumor may require dissection up to the greater curvature of the stomach. Identification of avascular spaces prior to dividing the pedicles will reduce the risk of bleeding from these high-pressure vessels.

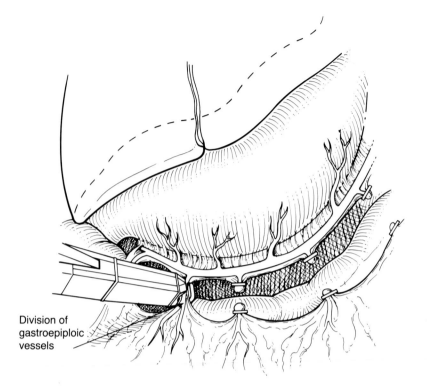

Division of
gastroepiploic
vessels

Figure 7–16. Division of smaller vascular pedicles can be accomplished with a stapling device. However, larger vessels such as the gastroepiploics are more secure if suture-ligated. Postoperative distention of the stomach should be avoided by nasogastric decompression or gastrostomy tube to avoid disruption of the vascular pedicles.

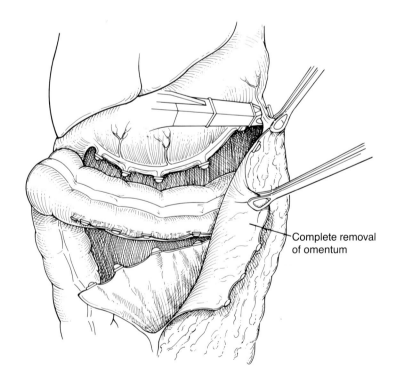

Complete removal
of omentum

Figure 7–17. Final dissection of the omentum involves division of the attachments at the hepatic and splenic flexures of the transverse colon. Ovarian cancer will often extend close to or into the hilum of the spleen. Excessive traction on the omentum while extending the dissection toward the spleen should be avoided. Splenic laceration during omentectomy is a major source of injury to this organ in gynecologic surgery.

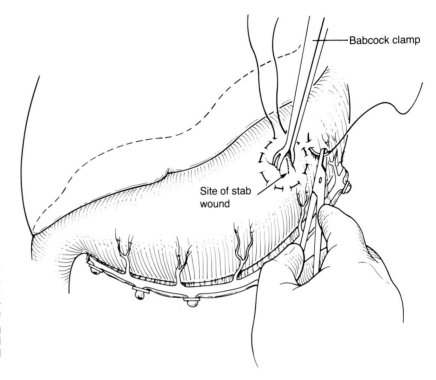

Figure 7-18. Gastrostomy drainage following extensive omental dissection or to palliate small bowel obstruction can be performed quickly and safely. A dependent and mobile site on the greater curvature of the stomach is identified. Two purse-string sutures of chromic suture are placed around the chosen site, which is elevated by a Babcock clamp.

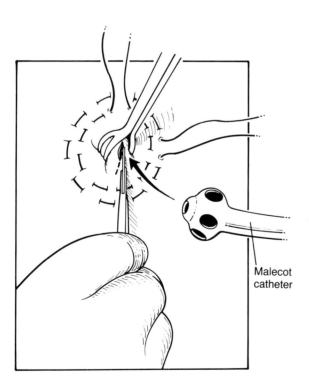

Figure 7-19. A stab wound is made in the middle of the purse string, and a large-bore drainage tube (28 to 32 French Malecot or mushroom catheter) is inserted.

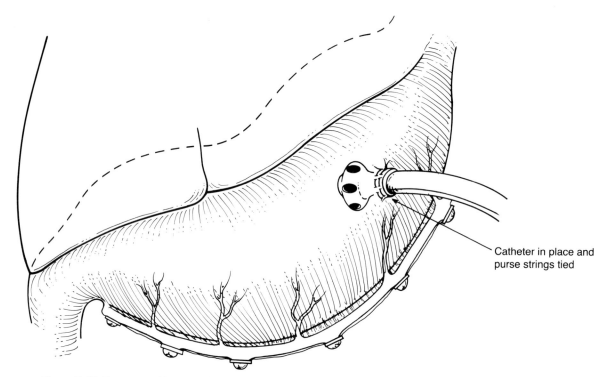

Catheter in place and
purse strings tied

Figure 7–20. The purse strings are tied down, and the tube is pulled back to rest against the stomach wall.

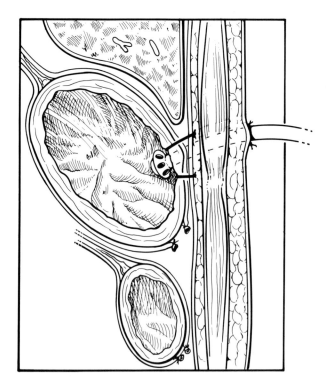

Figure 7–21. The distal end of the gastrostomy tube is brought out through a separate stab wound lateral to the incision. The insertion site on the stomach is tacked to the anterior abdominal wall to prevent leakage of gastric contents when the tube is eventually removed.

PART III. REVERSE HYSTERECTOMY

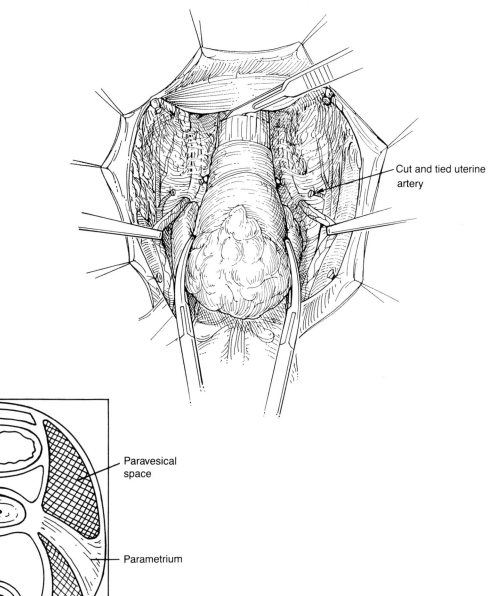

Cut and tied uterine artery

Paravesical space

Parametrium

Pararectal space

Figure 7–22. The procedure up to this point is similar to that shown in Figures 7–1 through 7–8. The ureter is retracted lateral and the uterine artery is divided medial to the ureter. The junction of the vagina and cervix has been identified by palpation, and the vagina is incised along its anterior aspect.

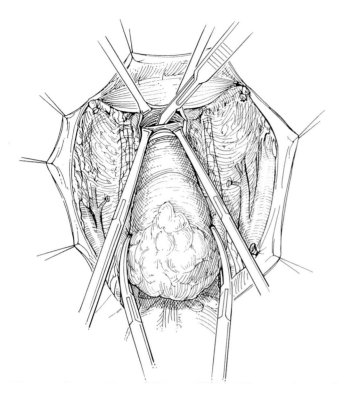

Figure 7-23. The posterior vagina is incised and the mucosal edges are grasped with Kocher clamps. The vaginal angles are ligated.

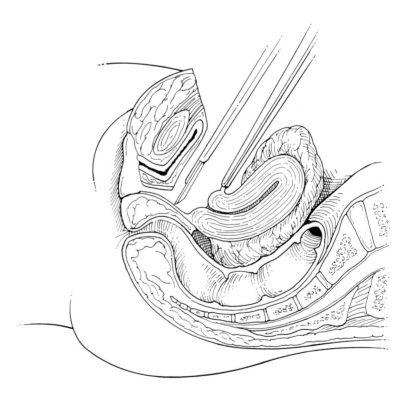

Figure 7-24. Lateral view depicting the incision of the posterior vaginal wall.

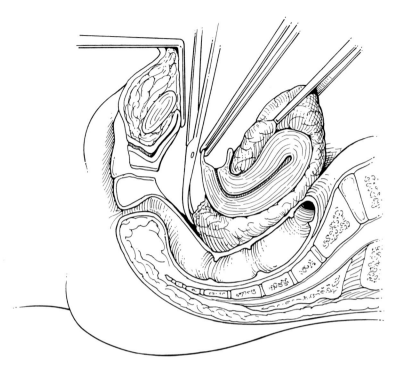

Figure 7–25. The posterior vaginal wall is grasped and retracted cephalad. The uterus can now be sharply dissected off of the rectosigmoid.

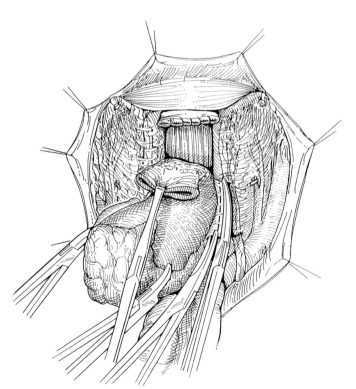

Figure 7–26. The cardinal ligaments and uterosacral ligaments are divided close to the uterus.

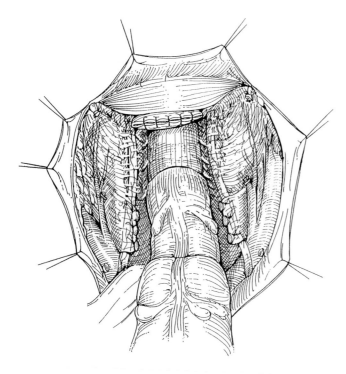

Figure 7–27. The pelvis is shown following removal of the specimen. The vaginal cuff is sutured closed.

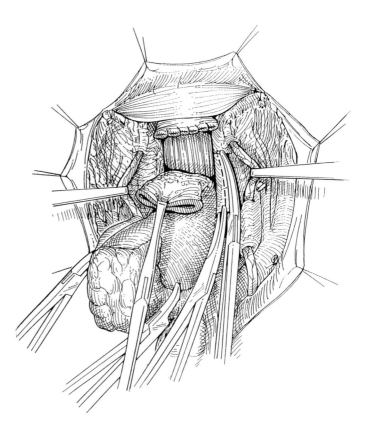

Figure 7–28. If removal of the sigmoid is indicated, the procedure is expanded to mobilize the ureters laterally to expose the rectal pillars. This tissue is divided, mobilizing the rectosigmoid.

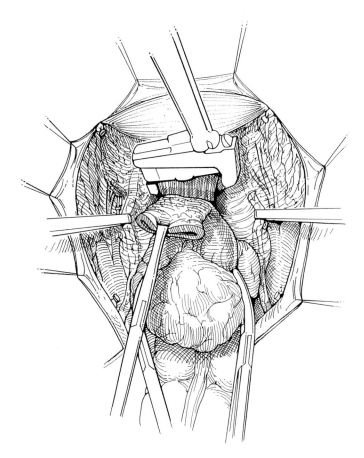

Figure 7–29. The rectum is divided with an end-stapling device. The ureters must be well visualized and retracted laterally.

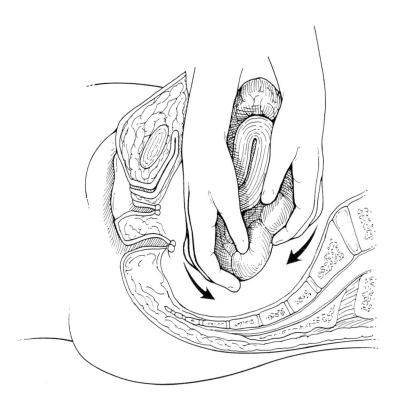

Figure 7–30. The sigmoid has been transected at its cephalad end. The specimen is dissected off of the sacrum from a cephalad and caudad direction. The sigmoid can be reanastomosed with an end-to-end anastomosis stapler, or an end sigmoid colostomy can be done. In patients with no visible remaining tumor, we prefer the former.

REFERENCES

1. Blythe JG, Wahl TP: Debulking surgery: Does it increase the quality of survival? Gynecol Oncol 14:396–408, 1982.
2. Chen SS, Bochner R: Assessment of morbidity and mortality in primary cytoreductive surgery for advanced ovarian carcinoma. Gynecol Oncol 20:190–195, 1985.
3. Delgado G, Oram DH, Petrilli ES: Stage III epithelial ovarian cancer: The role of maximal surgical reduction. Gynecol Oncol 18:293–298, 1984.
4. Griffiths CT, Parker LM, Fuller AF Jr: Role of cytoreductive surgical treatment in the management of advanced ovarian cancer. Cancer Treat Rep 63:235–240, 1979.
5. Hacker NF, Berek JS, Lagasse LD, et al: Primary cytoreductive surgery for epithelial ovarian cancer. Obstet Gynecol 61:413–420, 1983.
6. Morris M, Gershenson DM, Burke TW, et al: Splenectomy in gynecologic oncology: Indications, complications, and technique. Gynecol Oncol 43:118–122, 1991.
7. Neijt JP, Aartsen EJ, Bouma J, et al: Cytoreductive surgery with or without preceding chemotherapy in ovarian cancer. Primary Chemotherapy in Cancer Medicine 201:217–223, 1985.
8. Omura GA, Bundy BN, Berek JS, et al: Randomized trial of cyclophosphamide plus cisplatin with or without doxorubicin in ovarian carcinoma: A Gynecologic Oncology Group study. J Clin Oncol 7:457–465, 1989.
9. Wharton JT, Herson J: Surgery for common epithelial tumors of the ovary. Cancer 48:582–589, 1981.
10. Wils J, Blijham G, Naus A, et al: Primary or delayed debulking surgery and chemotherapy consisting of cisplatin, doxorubicin, and cyclophosphamide in Stage III–IV epithelial ovarian carcinoma. J Clin Oncol 4:1068–1073, 1986.

8

Extraperitoneal Approaches to Para-aortic Nodes

Many gynecologic oncologists will routinely perform limited staging procedures on patients with advanced stage (II through IV) cervical cancer in order to place patients on institutional or national group protocols such as that of the Gynecologic Oncology Group. The status of the para-aortic nodes should be known prior to initiation of treatment in order to plan appropriate modalities, such as extended field irradiation or concomitant chemotherapy.[1, 3, 6] Several investigators have noted a decreased morbidity, particularly regarding late small bowel injury, when an extraperitoneal approach for removal of para-aortic nodes is used as opposed to a transperitoneal approach.[2, 7]

POTENTIAL PROBLEM AREAS

Pathophysiologic changes from the procedures include possible formation of a lymphocyst and later herniation of bowel through presumably intact peritoneum. One point of caution: If the peritoneum is entered by either of the two approaches described below, it must be closed immediately. Often, in very thin patients, the peritoneum is entered, and a rent is not recognized. This event is particularly likely with "sunrise" incisions, and the peritoneum must be carefully inspected prior to closure.[5]

The midline incision, as noted in Chapter 4, may be used as an extraperitoneal approach and simply extended more cephalad for access to the para-aortic nodes. However, this incision is in the middle of the pelvic irradiation field, and some radiation oncologists are reluctant to begin radiation therapy until wound healing is complete. The two approaches described in this chapter can be used with patients who need timely initiation of irradiation.

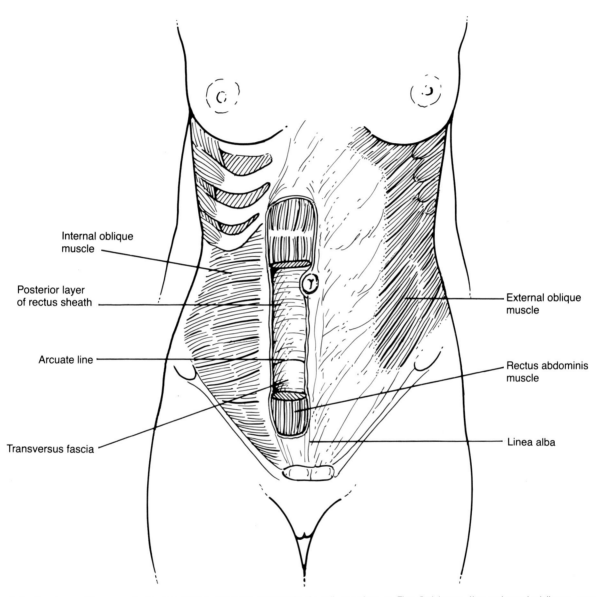

Figure 8–1. *Anatomy.* The muscle layers of the anterior abdominal wall are shown. The first layer, the external oblique, courses caudad and medially in an oblique fashion to the linea alba. Deep to the external oblique is the internal oblique, which courses from lateral to medial in an upward oblique fashion.

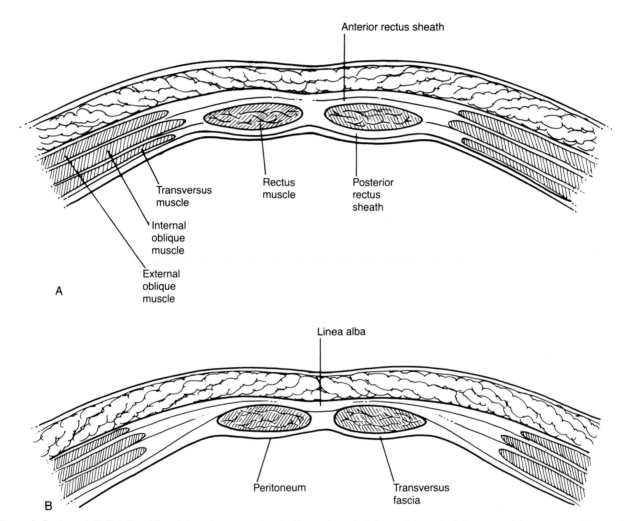

Figure 8–2. *A* and *B*, Relationship of the strap muscles to the external oblique, internal oblique, and transversus. Above the semilunar (arcuate) line, a posterior sheath is present. Below the semilunar (arcuate) line, the posterior sheath is absent.

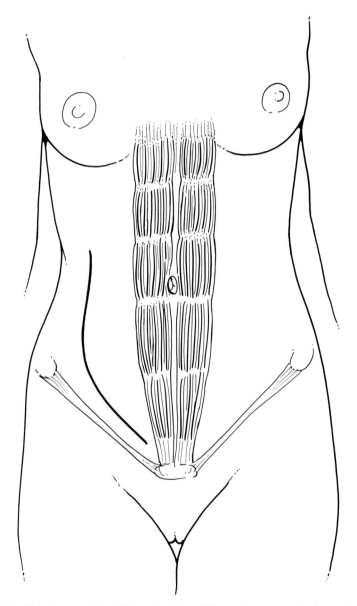

Figure 8–3. *The J-shaped incision.* This is a modified Gibson incision. Although some prefer to perform this on the left side,[2] we prefer to use the right-sided approach. Because the vena cava lies posterior and lateral to the aorta, the right-sided approach gives better access to the precaval nodes. The incision begins just medial to the pubic tubercle. It extends just parallel to and 2 cm above the inguinal ligament and 2 cm medial to the iliac crest, extending several centimeters cephalad to the umbilicus for adequate exposure of the para-aortic nodes.[4]

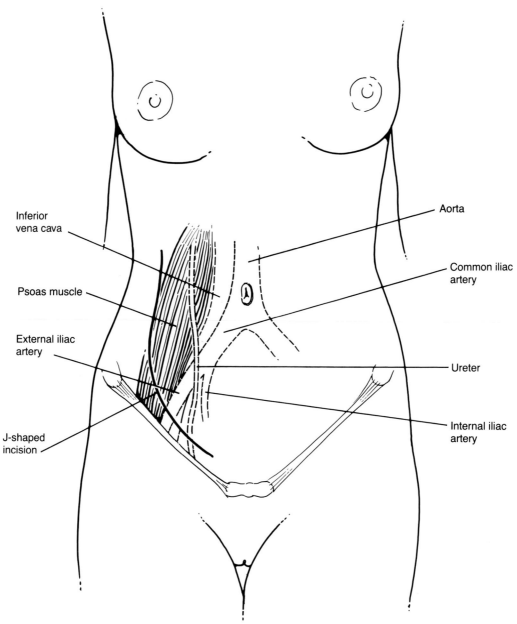

Figure 8–4. The J-shaped incision in relation to deeper structures, the ureter, iliac vessels, and great vessels. The blood supply to the anterior abdominal wall has been described in Chapter 4. When using the J-shaped incision, care must be taken to avoid the lateral anastomotic branches of the deep circumflex and musculophrenic arteries and associated veins.

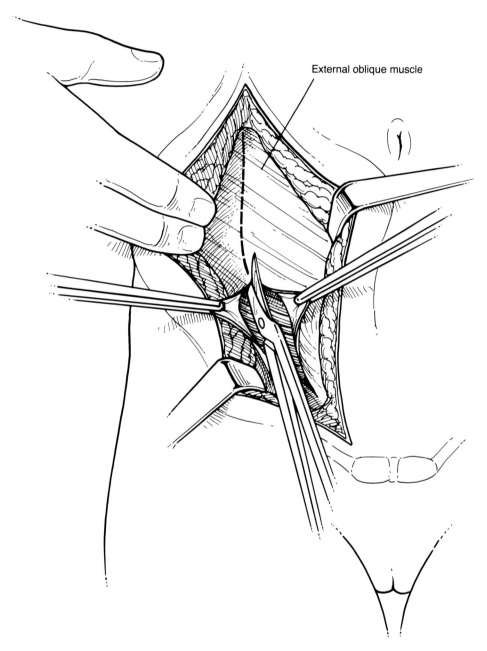

External oblique muscle

Figure 8–5. The J-shaped incision has been carried down to the fascia of the external oblique. The external oblique is sharply incised with the scissors as noted here, or with a knife, and the incision is carried from the pubic tubercle to above the umbilicus.

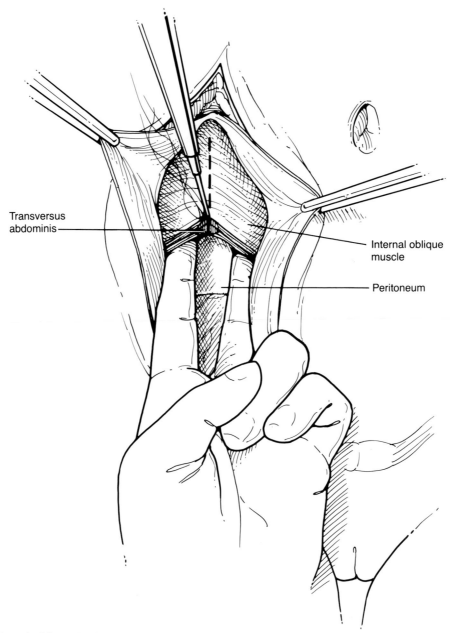

Transversus
abdominis

Internal oblique
muscle

Peritoneum

Figure 8–6. The external oblique fascia is shown retracted with small clamps. The internal oblique and transversus are then sectioned. The fingers of the operator push the peritoneum medial and posterior while these two muscles are sharply incised. The Bovie is used to transect these muscles, with the fingers of the operator protecting the underlying peritoneum.

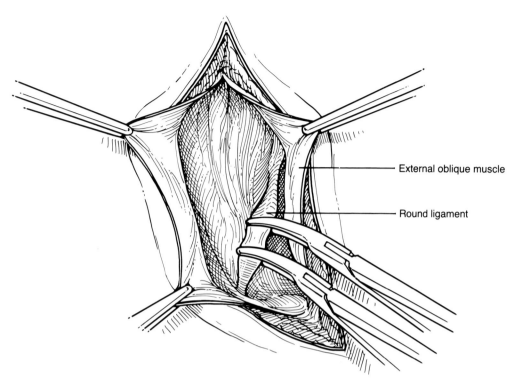

Figure 8–7. The external oblique is retracted with clamps. The internal oblique and transversus have been previously sectioned. The round ligament is isolated, clamped, sectioned, and tied extraperitoneally. A suture ligature should be used for hemostatic control. Sectioning the round ligament will offer more complete exposure of the para-aortic nodes. Often, the deep inferior epigastric vessels are sectioned and tied in order to avoid injury during manipulation of the peritoneum.

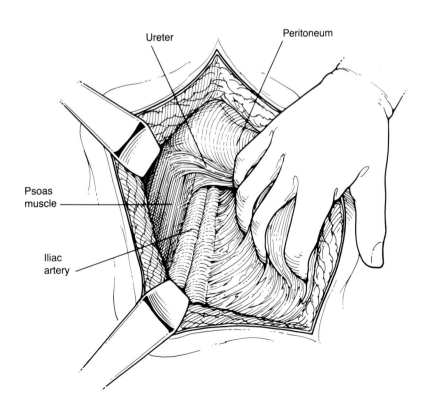

Figure 8–8. With the round ligament sectioned, the peritoneum is bluntly dissected by the hand of the operator. The psoas muscle is palpated, as is the external iliac artery lying medial to the psoas. The peritoneum is gently swept from lateral and caudad to medial and cephalad. This maneuver will easily expose the psoas muscle and the pelvic vessels. The ureter will remain on the medial leaf of the retracted peritoneum.

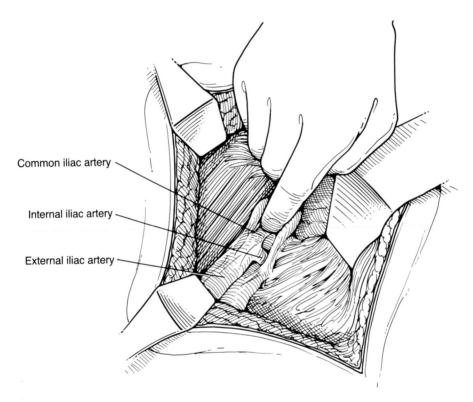

Common iliac artery

Internal iliac artery

External iliac artery

Figure 8–9. Once the pelvic vessels have been exposed, with the peritoneum retracted medially, the finger of the operator is placed over the external iliac vessels. In a gentle motion, the finger is swept caudad from the area of the inguinal ligament to cephalad along the external iliac artery, the common iliac artery, and the aorta in order to remove some of the loose areolar tissue over these vessels. In order to avoid bleeding, the finger should be kept directly over these arteries.

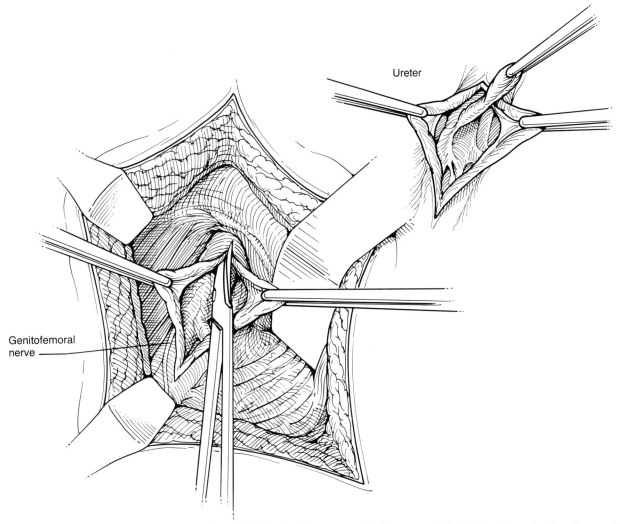

Figure 8–10. The extraperitoneal space on the right side has been completely exposed. An incision is made directly over the external iliac artery. It may be carried cephalad to the level of just above the inferior mesenteric artery and caudad to the level of the inguinal ligament. Note that the ureter is retracted medially, and the genitofemoral nerve is lateral to the vessels. Pelvic and para-aortic nodes are moved in the usual fashion. When removing para-aortic nodes, small clips should be used prior to any sectioning in order to avoid oozing from small arteries or veins.

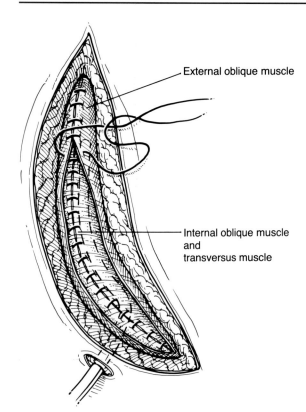

External oblique muscle

Internal oblique muscle
and
transversus muscle

Figure 8-11. The nodes have been removed. The transversus and internal oblique muscles are closed with running suture of delayed absorbable suture (Maxon or PDS II). The external oblique muscle is then closed separately with the same interrupted delayed absorbable suture. A Blake or Jackson-Pratt (JP) closed drainage system is placed posterior to the transversus muscle in the area of the vessels and brought out through a separate stab wound in the skin to provide drainage from the pelvic node area. It is left in place for 3 to 5 days, depending on the extent of pelvic node dissection and the drainage. The skin can be closed with staples.

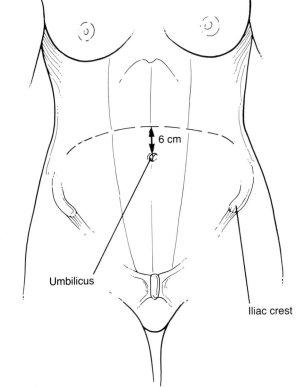

6 cm

Umbilicus

Iliac crest

Figure 8-12. Because the main objective of the staging procedure is to access the status of the para-aortic nodes, we prefer to use the "sunrise" incision. In the center, this incision is approximately 6 cm above the umbilicus.[4, 5] The bifurcation of the aorta can often be assessed by computed tomographic (CT) scan preoperatively by placing a radiopaque object at the level of the umbilicus. Thus, the site of the incision can be varied. The incision is carried laterally in a downward fashion to the level of the iliac crests. In thin patients, a unilateral incision, usually done on the right side, can be used and adequate exposure to para-aortic nodes on both sides can be obtained. In the event of palpable, bulky disease in the lower common iliac or pelvic nodes, the incision can be extended in a caudad fashion to remove the nodes.

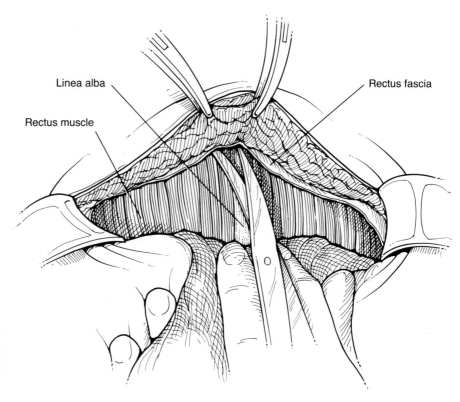

Figure 8–13. The fascia has been incised in a transverse manner. The rectus muscles are dissected free of their attachments from the anterior-lying fascia cephalad and caudad in the midline. A Bovie may be used instead of the scissors.

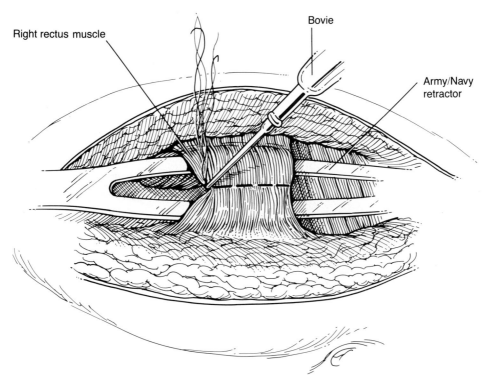

Figure 8–14. An Army-Navy retractor is inserted posterior to the rectus muscle. The right rectus muscle is sectioned with the Bovie. Because the deep epigastric vessels lie in the middle and posterior to the rectus muscle, there is no need to attempt to isolate them laterally. The vessels are small in this area, and bleeding can usually be controlled with the Bovie or ties.

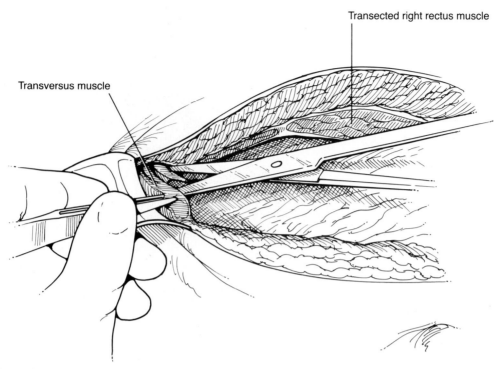

Figure 8–15. The rectus muscle has been transected. The transversus muscle is noted laterally. It is incised with the scissors. A Bovie may be used instead of the scissors.

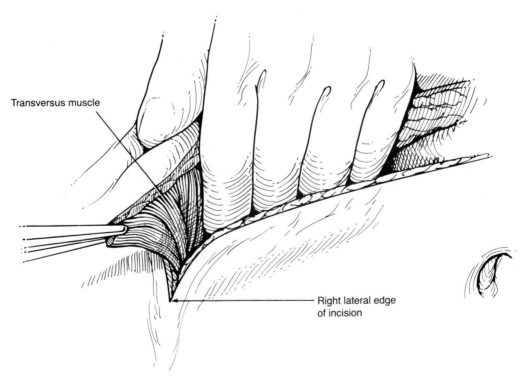

Figure 8–16. The peritoneum is retracted medially and cephalad by the hand of the operator. The incision into the transversus is carried more caudad and laterally to complete the transection of this muscle without entering the peritoneum.

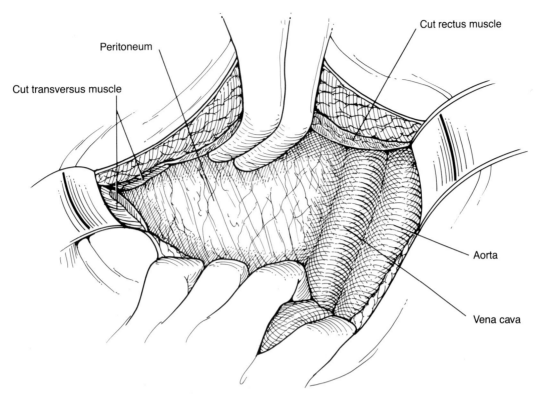

Figure 8–17. The transversus muscle has been almost completely incised. The fingers of the operator ''stretch'' the wound in order to ensure adequate exposure so that the hand of the operator can be inserted into the incision.

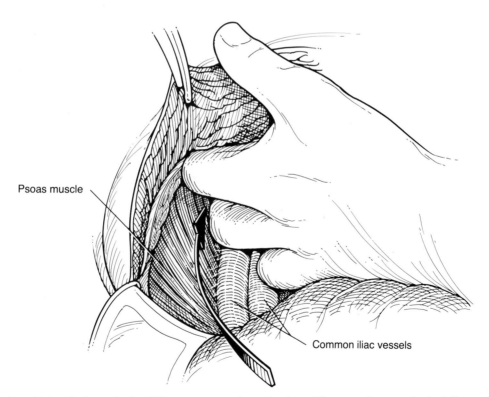

Figure 8–18. The hand is inserted caudad until the psoas muscle and external iliac vessels are palpated. The peritoneum is then bluntly dissected from caudad and lateral to cephalad and medial, separating it from the underlying common iliac vessels until the aorta and vena cava are exposed. A self-retaining retractor may be inserted.

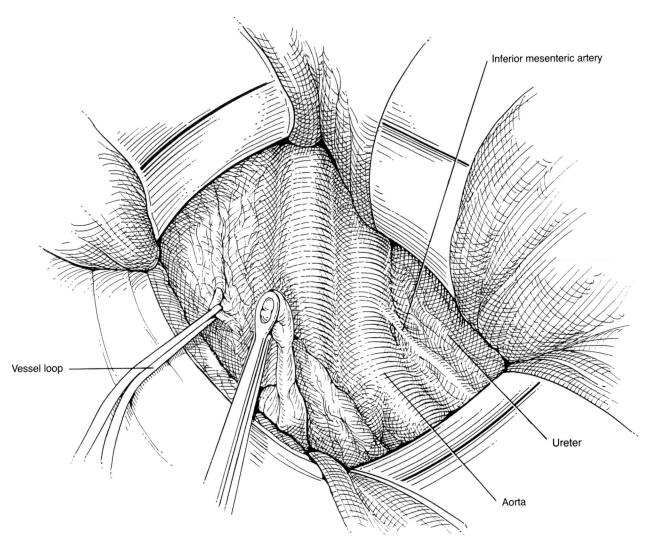

Figure 8–19. A vessel loop pulls the ureter lateral to avoid injury. The aorta and vena cava are seen medially. Also identified are the ovarian vessels, which course lateral to the ureter.

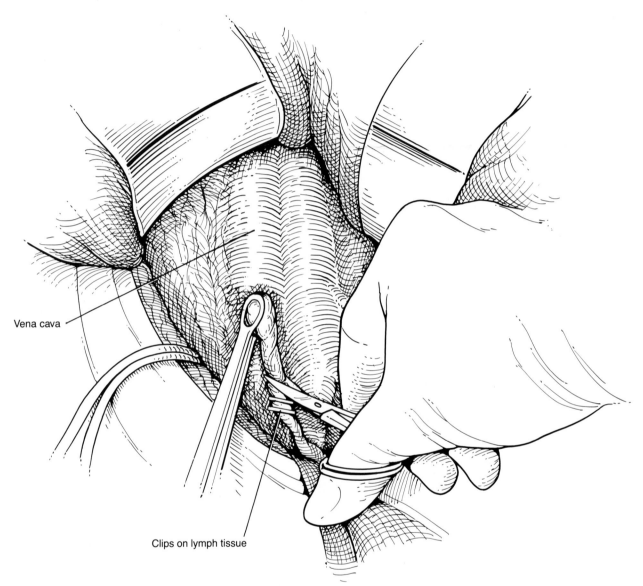

Vena cava

Clips on lymph tissue

Figure 8–20. The fat containing the lymph tissue over the vena cava is grasped with Singley forceps. A right-angle clamp is inserted posterior to the fat pad and anterior to the vena cava. This is done at the level of the mid-portion of the common iliac artery on the right. Two large vascular clips are placed at this level. The fat pad is then transected. With gentle traction, small clips are utilized on either side of the fat pad to remove it completely from the underlying vena cava. Often the para-aortic nodes can be removed from this incision from the level of the midcommon left iliac vessels to the inferior mesenteric artery. However, if exposure is difficult, the left rectus muscle can be transected and the peritoneum mobilized from the left side, as previously described.

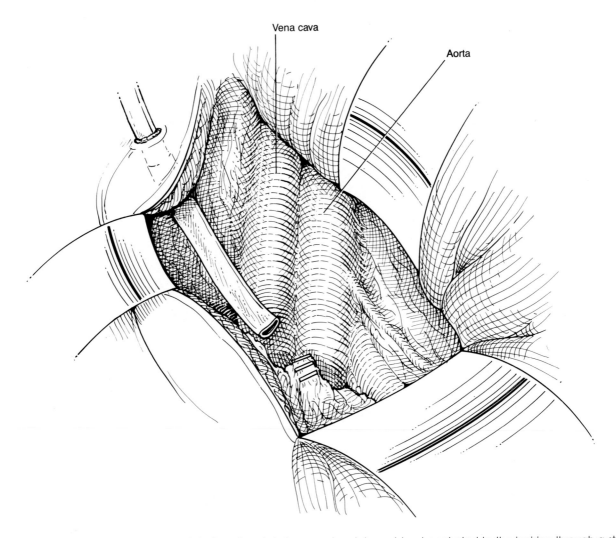

Vena cava

Aorta

Figure 8–21. With node dissection completed, a closed drainage system is brought out cephalad to the incision through a stab wound. The Blake or Jackson-Pratt (JP) drain is placed deep in the extraperitoneal space. The fascia and skin are closed in the usual manner.

REFERENCES

1. Averette HE, Dudan RC, Ford JH Jr.: Exploratory celiotomy for surgical staging of cervical cancer. Am J Obstet Gynecol 113:1090, 1972.
2. Berman ML, Lagasse LD, Watring WG, et al: The operative evaluation of patients with cervical cancer by an extraperitoneal approach. Obstet Gynecol 50:658, 1977.
3. Delgado G, Bundy BN, Fowler WC, et al: A prospective surgical pathological study of Stage I squamous carcinoma of the cervix: A Gynecologic Oncology Group Study. Gynecol Oncol 35:314, 1989.
4. Gallup DG: Extraperitoneal and transperitoneal approaches for removal of retroperitoneal pelvic and paraaortic lymph nodes. In *Te Linde's Operative Gynecology Updates* (Published by JB Lippincott, Philadelphia), 1(8):1–14, 1993.
5. Gallup DG, King LA, Messing MJ, Talledo OE: Paraaortic lymph node sampling by means of an extraperitoneal approach with a supraumbilical transverse "sunrise" incision. Am J Obstet Gynecol 169:307, 1993.
6. Piver MS, Barlow JJ: Paraaortic lymphadenectomy in staging patients with advanced local cervical cancer. Obstet Gynecol 43:544, 1974.
7. Weiser EB, Bundy BN, Hoskins WJ, et al: Extraperitoneal versus transperitoneal selective paraaortic lymphadenectomy in the pretreatment surgical staging of advanced cervical carcinoma: A Gynecologic Oncology Group Study. Gynecol Oncol 33:283, 1989.

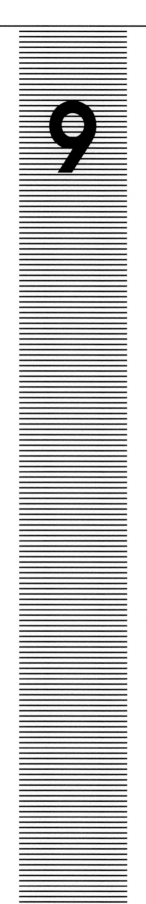

9

Transperitoneal Approach to the Para-aortic Lymph Nodes

Mark J. Messing, M.D.

Surgical evaluation of the retroperitoneal para-aortic lymph nodes is a commonly performed procedure in the management of gynecologic malignancies. The incidence of para-aortic lymph node metastases varies with different gynecologic malignancies. Most gynecologic oncologists limit the para-aortic lymph node evaluation to the lymphatic tissue overlying the vena cava and aorta from their bifurcation up to the level of the duodenum.

The surgical approach to the retroperitoneum surrounding the aorta and vena cava can be accomplished by (1) a direct approach via the root of the small bowel mesentery or (2) by reflection of the left or right colon. The advantage of the direct approach is less associated dissection of the intestine and ureter. Disadvantages include more difficulty in approaching the left para-aortic lymph nodes and possibly more risk from bowel adhesions and subsequent injury should later adjunctive radiation therapy be administered. The lateral approach, by reflecting the colon, allows a more exposed view of the great vessels, ureters, and the lymph-bearing areas. More extensive mobilization of the colon can result in bleeding or potential injury to the ureters.

The indications for para-aortic lymph node evaluation in gynecologic malignancies are still evolving. Cancer of the uterus and ovary are surgically staged diseases, and evaluation of lymph-bearing areas is now included in the staging system. Indications for para-aortic lymph node evaluation in ovarian cancer include those patients with disease that appears limited to the ovaries or pelvis.[7] Retroperitoneal disease would place these women in a higher disease stage and potentially would alter therapy. Evaluation of para-aortic lymph nodes in patients undergoing second-look laparotomy for ovarian cancer is also standard practice.[1]

Controversy still exists over the indications for para-aortic lymph node evaluation in endometrial cancer. The incidence of para-aortic node involvement increases with tumor grade, depth of myometrial invasion, presence of extrauterine disease, involvement of the cervix, vascular space involvement, and positive cytology.[3, 5] About one third of patients with pelvic lymph node involvement will have para-aortic lymph node metastases.[3] Morbidity from para-aortic evaluation in endometrial cancer patients may be higher owing to other constitutional risk factors such as age, obesity, diabetes, and other medical problems.[5]

Cancer of the cervix is clinically staged, and patients with advanced local disease are typically evaluated with various imaging methods to detect metastatic disease. Surgical staging of advanced cervix cancer patients has shown that the incidence of para-aortic metastases can be high. The transperitoneal approach has been criticized in this group because the subsequent use of para-aortic radiation is associated with a higher risk of complications (small bowel obstruction) than in patients who underwent extraperitoneal lymph node staging.[6] Patients undergoing primary exploration for early stage cervix cancer should have palpation of the para-aortic area prior to radical hysterectomy to evaluate for clinically suspicious nodes. Occult metastases in stage IB cervical cancer occur in 5 per cent of cases, the incidence increasing up to 35 per cent with larger tumors.[2, 4] If metastatic disease is discovered at the time of pelvic lymphadenectomy, evaluation of the para-aortic lymph nodes would be warranted.

PATHOPHYSIOLOGY

Extensive mobilization of the viscera from the retroperitoneum for lymph node evaluation appears to be a well-tolerated procedure. Morbidity is usually described as extended operative time, postoperative ileus, and the potential for intraoperative hemorrhage. Obese patients with underlying medical problems need to be individually assessed for their ability to tolerate an extended lymph node staging procedure. A preoperative mechanical intestinal preparation will deflate the bowel and allow for easier exposure. Postoperative ileus can occur following a high dissection and mobilization of the duodenum. Nasogastric decompression is routine in these patients until intestinal activity has returned.

POTENTIAL PROBLEM AREAS

The proximity of the great vessels, ureter, and ovarian vessels makes exposure and identification of the retroperitoneal structures essential for safe dissection. Proper exposure and isolation of the ureter will prevent injury should bleeding hinder exposure. The major lymphatic tissue on the right overlies the vena cava and is easily separated from the vessel. A small vein may arise near the bifurcation and can be avulsed during the dissection, resulting in brisk bleeding. Repair requires excellent exposure with isolation of the ureter from the field. Repair with a permanent suture (5-0 polypropylene) on a vascular needle will usually suffice. The left para-aortic lymphatic chain lies lateral and somewhat behind the aorta. Small lumbar branches can cause troublesome bleeding if vascular clips are not placed during the dissection. Additionally, the inferior mesenteric artery arises approximately 4 cm above the bifurcation. Care should be taken to preserve this vessel.

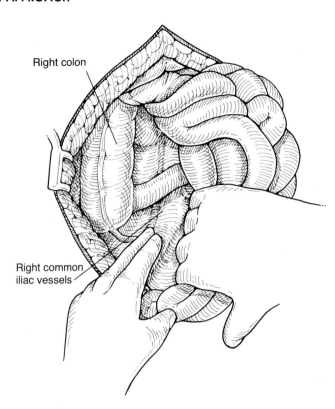

Right colon

Right common
iliac vessels

Figure 9–1. The abdomen has been opened through a vertical midline incision that extends around the umbilicus. The small bowel is elevated out of the pelvis, and the base of the mesentery is placed on tension. The right pelvic vessels are palpated, and the ureter is identified through the peritoneum.

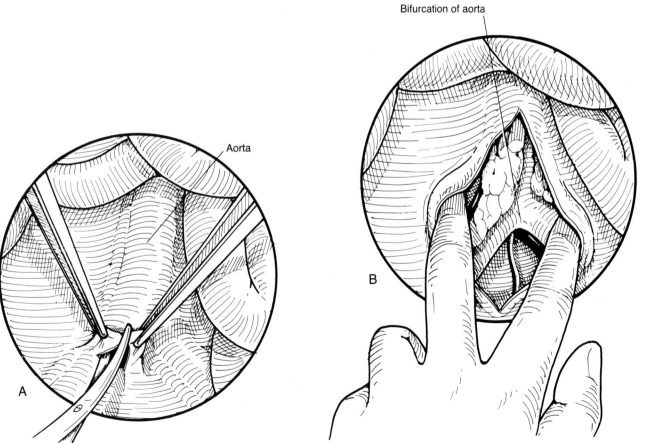

Bifurcation of aorta

Aorta

A

B

Figure 9–2. *A,* The peritoneum is elevated over the right common iliac artery and is incised. The incision should be started cephalad to where the ureter crosses this vessel to avoid injury. By keeping the mesentery on tension, it can be elevated off of the vessels as it is incised. The incision can be carried as high as the ligament of Treitz. *B,* Blunt dissection can be used to separate the peritoneum from the underlying retroperitoneal structures. The dissection continues laterally to mobilize the ureter from the vessels and psoas muscle, while keeping it attached to the peritoneum.

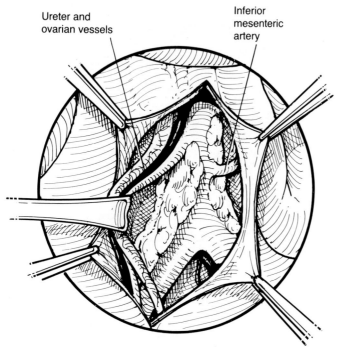

Ureter and
ovarian vessels

Inferior
mesenteric
artery

Figure 9–3. The retroperitoneum is exposed by retraction on the incised peritoneal edges. Small Deaver retractors can be placed on either side of the incision to open the space, keeping the small bowel out of the field. An alternative is the use of traction sutures on the peritoneal edges.

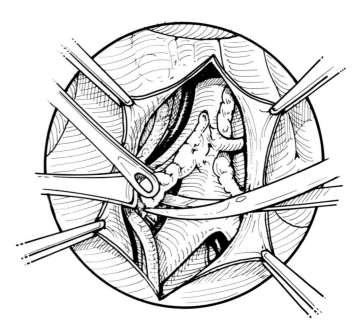

Figure 9–4. The dissection is started over the right common iliac artery. The lymphatic tissue is elevated and the caudal end clipped and divided. The ureter and ovarian vessels are retracted laterally to avoid injury.

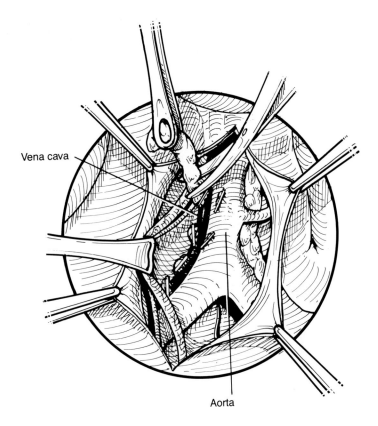

Vena cava

Aorta

Figure 9–5. The specimen is dissected in a cephalad direction. Hemostatic clips are used on either side of the developing pedicle as it is mobilized and divided. Dissection off of the vena cava can usually be done bluntly because there is rarely firm adhesion of normal tissue to the vein. Inflammatory or malignant nodes may be more densely adherent and require meticulous sharp dissection. When the most cephalad extent of the dissection is reached, the pedicle is clipped and divided.

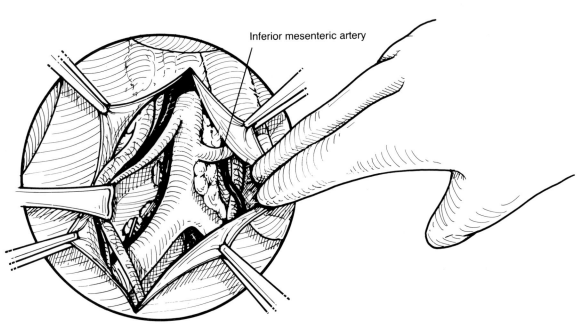

Inferior mesenteric artery

Figure 9–6. The left common iliac and left para-aortic lymph nodes can be removed through the same incision. Blunt dissection is again used to mobilize the peritoneum from the underlying vessels, and the ureter is mobilized laterally.

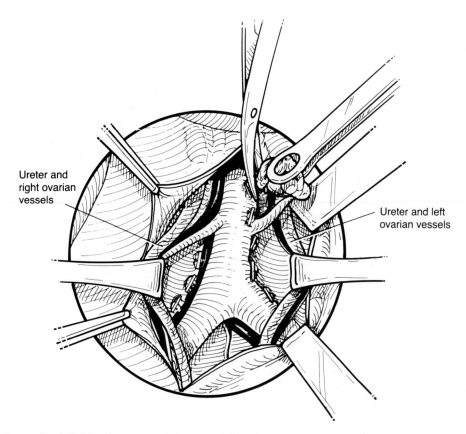

Ureter and
right ovarian
vessels

Ureter and left
ovarian vessels

Figure 9–7. Dissection on the left side also proceeds in a caudal to cephalad direction. Hemostatic clips are used on the lateral and medial margins of dissection. Care should be taken to avoid injury to lumbar branches because the lymph nodes tend to be more posterior to the vessel on the left. The inferior mesenteric artery arises approximately 4 cm above the bifurcation.

REFLECTION OF THE RIGHT COLON

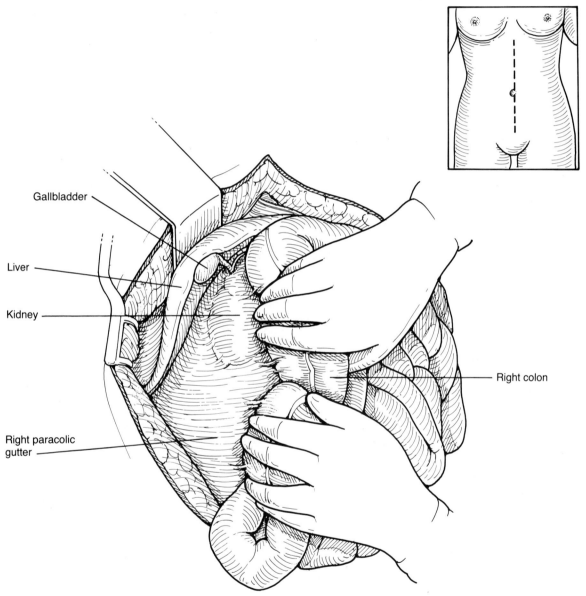

Gallbladder

Liver

Kidney

Right paracolic gutter

Right colon

Figure 9–8. The abdomen is opened through a vertical midline incision that extends around the umbilicus. The right paracolic gutter is exposed by medial traction on the ascending colon.

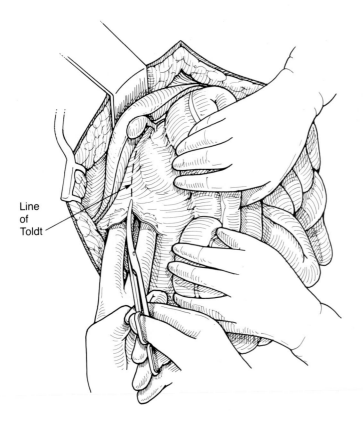

Line
of
Toldt

Figure 9–9. The peritoneum overlying the psoas muscle is incised at the pelvic brim and extended cephalad along the line of Toldt (''white line''). During this incision, blunt dissection will help elevate the peritoneum off the psoas muscle. The incision can be extended cephalad to the hepatic flexure of the colon.

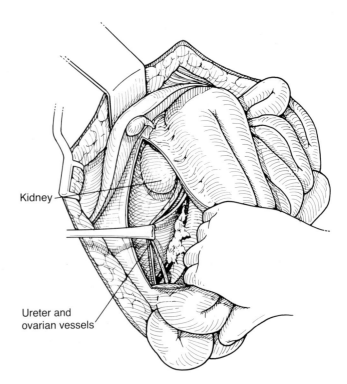

Kidney

Ureter and
ovarian vessels

Figure 9–10. The colon is reflected medially with blunt and sharp dissection. The ureter and ovarian vessels will be identified attached to the reflected peritoneum. These structures can be freed from the peritoneum and retracted laterally as shown or left attached, depending on the exposure required and the anticipated cephalad extent of the lymph node dissection. Further mobilization of the colon will expose the vena cava and aorta.

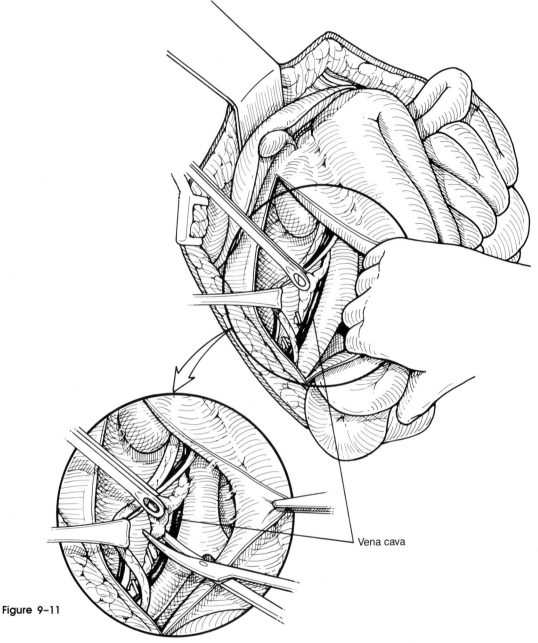

Figure 9–11

Vena cava

Figures 9–11 and 9–12. The lymphatic tissue is divided over the right common iliac artery, and dissection proceeds cephalad. Hemostatic clips are placed lateral and medial to the dissection. With this exposure, dissection can proceed to the third portion of the duodenum. The origin of the ovarian vessels must be identified, and the ureter must be visualized along its entire course. Access to the left para-aortic lymphatics is difficult from a right-sided approach because the lymph nodes lie lateral and posterior to the aorta.

Illustration continued on following page

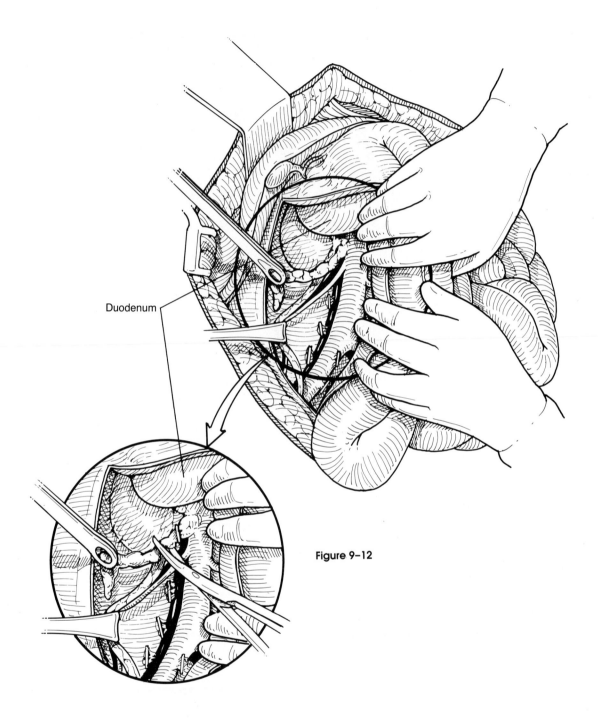

Duodenum

Figure 9–12

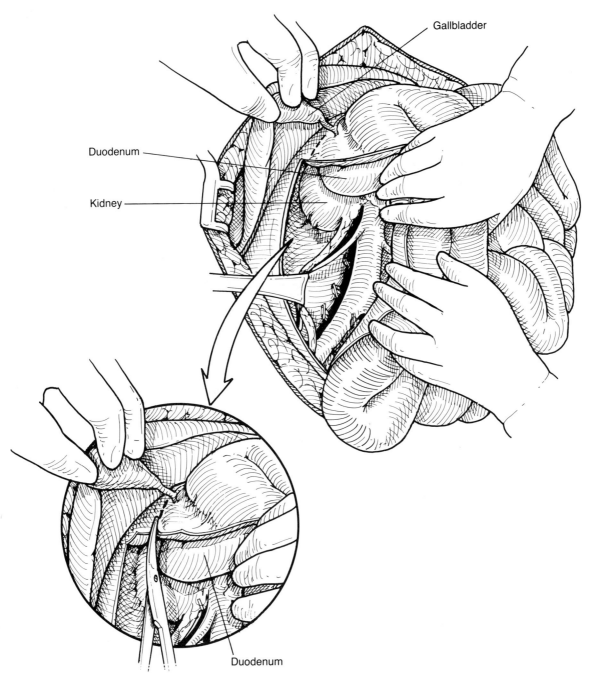

Gallbladder

Duodenum

Kidney

Duodenum

Figure 9–13. Access to lymph nodes at the level of the duodenum can be obtained with the Kocher maneuver, which reflects the duodenum medially. The peritoneal incision is carried cephalad to fully mobilize the right colon from the hepatic flexure. The peritoneum along the second portion of the duodenum is incised. Using blunt dissection, the first and second portions of the duodenum are mobilized medially. The common bile duct and pancreatic duct enter the second portion of the duodenum posteromedially.

REFLECTION OF THE LEFT COLON

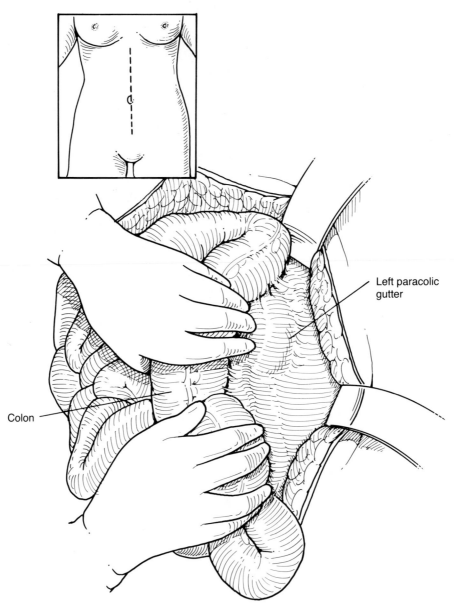

Left paracolic gutter

Colon

Figure 9–14. The abdomen has been opened through a vertical midline incision extending around the umbilicus. The left colon is retracted medially to expose the left paracolic gutter.

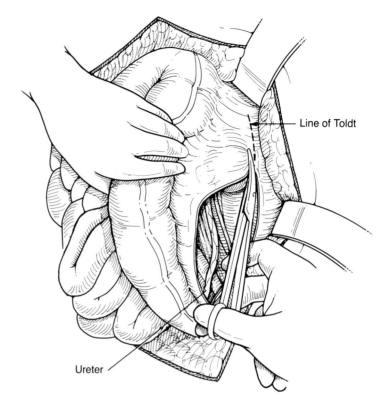

Line of Toldt

Ureter

Figure 9–15. The peritoneum overlying the psoas muscle is incised and the dissection is carried cephalad along the line of Toldt (''white line''). Blunt dissection with fingers elevates the peritoneum off the muscle and aids in exposure.

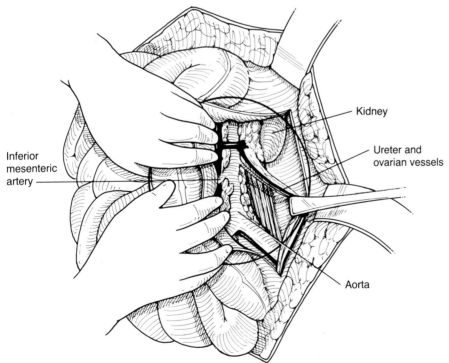

Inferior mesenteric artery

Kidney

Ureter and ovarian vessels

Aorta

Figure 9–16. Blunt and sharp dissection mobilizes the colon medially, exposing the ureter, ovarian vessels, and aorta. The ureter and ovarian vessels can be left attached to the peritoneum or mobilized laterally for better exposure.

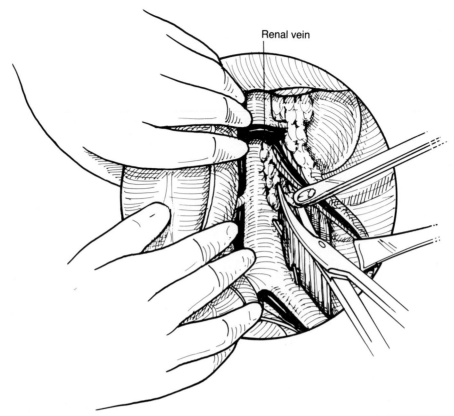

Renal vein

Figure 9–17. Dissection of the lymphatics begins at the common iliac artery and proceeds cephalad, utilizing hemostatic clips. The inferior mesenteric artery arises approximately 4 cm above the bifurcation and must be identified before proceeding more cephalad. The lymphatics tend to be more lateral and posterior to the aorta, and care should be taken to avoid injury to lumbar branches off of the aorta. Dissection of the right precaval lymphatics can be performed from the left side. The mesentery of the small bowel is elevated off of the vessels and allows access to the precaval lymphatics.

REFERENCES

1. Berek JS, Hacker NF, Lagasse LD, et al: Second-look laparotomy in stage 3 epithelial ovarian cancer: Clinical variables associated with disease status. Obstet Gynecol 64:207, 1984.
2. Coleman DL, Gallup DG, Wolcott HD, et al: Patterns of failure of bulky-barrel carcinomas of the cervix. Am J Obstet Gynecol 166:916, 1992.
3. Creasman WT, Morrow CP, Bundy BN, et al: Surgical pathologic spread patterns of endometrial cancer: A Gynecologic Oncology Group study. Cancer 60:2035, 1987.
4. Delgado G, Bundy BN, Fowler WC, et al: A prospective surgical pathological study of stage 1 squamous carcinoma of the cervix: A Gynecologic Oncology Group study. Gynecol Oncol 35:314, 1989.
5. Morrow CP, Bundy BN, Kumar RJ, et al: Relationship between surgical-pathological risk factors and outcome in clinical stages I and II carcinoma of the endometrium: A Gynecologic Oncology Group study. Gynecol Oncol 40:55, 1991.
6. Weiser EB, Bundy BN, Hoskins WJ, et al: Extraperitoneal versus transperitoneal selective paraaortic lymphadenectomy in the pretreatment surgical staging of advanced cervical carcinoma: A Gynecologic Oncology Group study. A Gynecol Oncol 33:283, 1989.
7. Young RC, Decker DG, Wharton JT, et al: Staging laparotomy in early ovarian cancer. JAMA 250:3072, 1983.

10

Total Pelvic
Exenteration

Total pelvic exenteration is a combination of well-established procedures employed in the treatment of a variety of pelvic cancers: (1) radical cystectomy; (2) radical hysterectomy with pelvic lymphadenectomy; and (3) abdominoperineal resection of the rectosigmoid. Inherent to the operation are urinary diversion following radical cystectomy and colostomy following abdominoperineal resection of the rectosigmoid.

Previously irradiated cancer of the cervix is the most common indication as well as the most suitable condition for this type of surgery. Other indications, determined by the extension and growth of the tumor, may include cancer of the ovary, uterus, vagina, vulva, or rectum and soft tissue sarcomas of the pelvis.

Preparation of the patient begins with appropriate diagnostic tests to rule out extension of the cancer beyond resectability. They include chest x-ray and computed tomography (CT) scan of the abdomen and pelvis with CT-guided needle biopsies of periaortic nodes when indicated. On occasion intravenous pyelography (IVP), barium enema, cystoscopy, and proctosigmoidoscopy may be useful, particularly if other than a total pelvic exenteration is being considered. Recently, magnetic resonance imaging (MRI) is gaining some interest because it may be possible to differentiate radiation fibrosis from cancer by this technique. The gastrointestinal tract is prepared for surgery with one of the common bowel preparation protocols. Assessment of the nutritional status should be performed 2 to 3 weeks prior to surgery. When appropriate, central hyperalimentation may be used preoperatively and is routinely used postoperatively.

Pelvic exenteration is a formidable procedure that taxes the patient severely as a result of anatomic and pathophysiologic changes associated with the operation. Indeed, the lack of popularity of this operation when Brunschwig first performed it in 1947 was due to loss of sexual function as well as an altered physiologic state in which the gastrointestinal tract and the urinary tract emptied through a common stoma (wet colostomy). The operative mortality, reported by Brunschwig at about 20 per cent, was also unacceptable. With the improvement in anesthesia, availability of central lines for monitoring, as well as hyperalimentation and refining of surgical techniques (including reconstructive procedures) to restore sexual function, this operation has become a mainstay of treatment in some patients with recurrent pelvic cancers. In recent years, urinary diversion by isolated loops of large or small bowel has been largely replaced by continent urinary pouches. This has resulted in better acceptance and improved body image by the patient undergoing this ultraradical procedure.

The technique described here is that of a total pelvic exenteration with excision of part of the vulva and perineum, commonly used in our patients with recurrent cervical cancers involving the distal vagina. However, several variations (less radical) are used, depending on location and extent of tumor. When in doubt, the more radical procedure should be performed.

The location of the stomas should be selected prior to surgery to ensure adequate fitting of the corresponding appliances. Alternate sites should also be considered. With the introduction of continent urinary pouches, selection of site is less critical.

POTENTIAL PROBLEM AREAS

A detailed description of potential problems is out of the scope of this atlas. We will simply categorize them as operative and postoperative. Such problems that may be encountered include (1) life-threatening hemorrhage during dissection of the pelvic side walls; (2) management of the enormous pelvic defect as a result of the extirpation of pelvic organs to prevent herniation of bowel and intestinal obstruction; (3) urinary and bowel fistulas following urinary diversion and entero-entero anastomosis can occur in the perioperative period or quite distant from the surgery; (4) stenosis of the ureter at the uretero-bowel anastomosis, causing chronic urinary infections with loss of renal function; and (5) sexual dysfunction. In the early years of performance of this procedure, the patient's ability to have sexual intercourse was lost. As a result, patients who otherwise may have benefited from the operation rejected it. With development of reconstructive techniques, this problem has been largely solved.

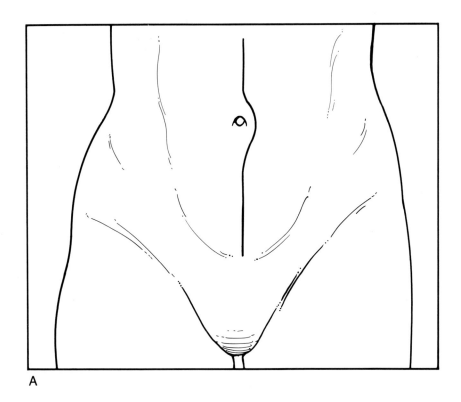

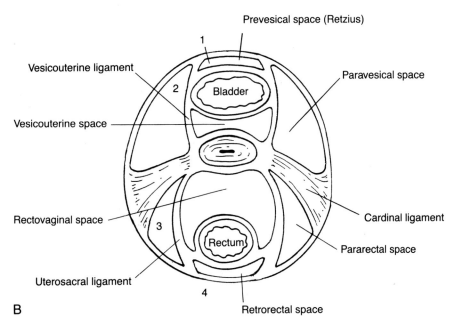

Prevesical space (Retzius)

Vesicouterine ligament

Vesicouterine space

Rectovaginal space

Uterosacral ligament

Paravesical space

Bladder

Cardinal ligament

Pararectal space

Rectum

Retrorectal space

B

Figure 10–1. *A* and *B*, The abdomen is opened through a vertical incision from symphysis pubis to halfway between xiphoid and umbilicus. A transverse incision is an alternative approach. A careful and systematic examination of the abdomen is carried out. We begin the exploration in the right upper quadrant with the right hemidiaphragm, liver, gallbladder, and kidney, followed by stomach, duodenum, and pancreas, left hemidiaphragm, spleen and left kidney, the colonic frame, and small intestines. Lymph nodes over the aorta and vena cava are evaluated with appropriate biopsies for frozen section. Attention is then turned to the pelvis, and a combined abdomino-recto-vaginal examination is very helpful in determining lateral extension of the cancer. Development of pelvic spaces—prevesical, retrorectal, paravesical, and pararectal—facilitates this step of the operation. Biopsies of the most lateral parametrium and pelvic floor are done. If their results are positive, the operation is abandoned. We have not had any long-term survivors when the proposed margin of resection or the pelvic floor has been involved with cancer.

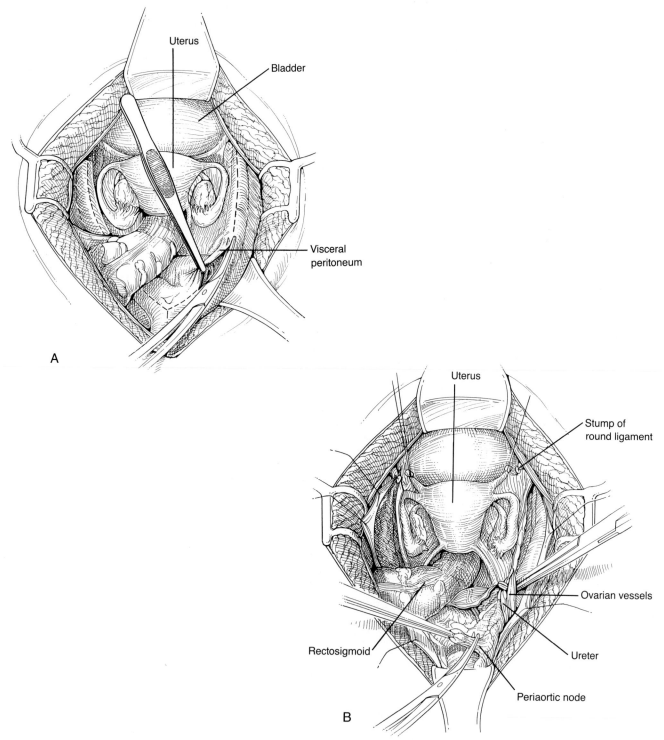

Figure 10–2. *A* and *B,* The peritoneum over the aortic bifurcation is opened and the incision extended on both sides to Poupart's ligaments. Nodes over the aorta and vena cava are sampled for frozen section. If they are positive for cancer, the operation is abandoned. While awaiting the results of the frozen section, the infundibulopelvic ligament is isolated and the ovarian vessels are ligated.

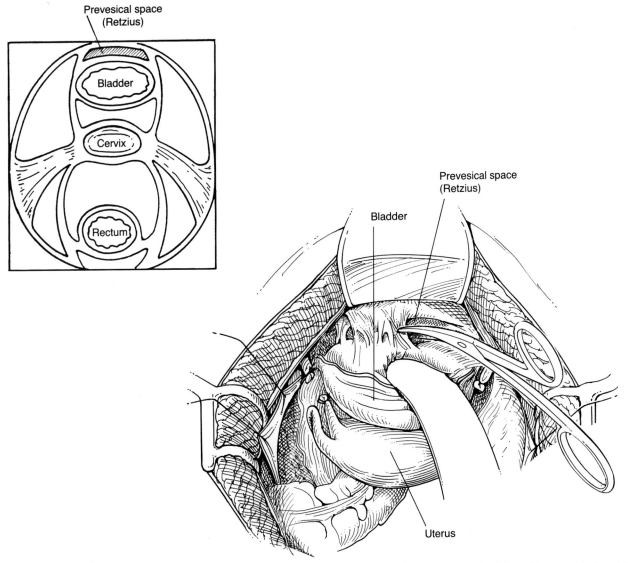

Figure 10-3. The pelvic spaces are developed. Anteriorly, the bladder and urethra are separated from the symphysis pubis, exposing the Retzius space.

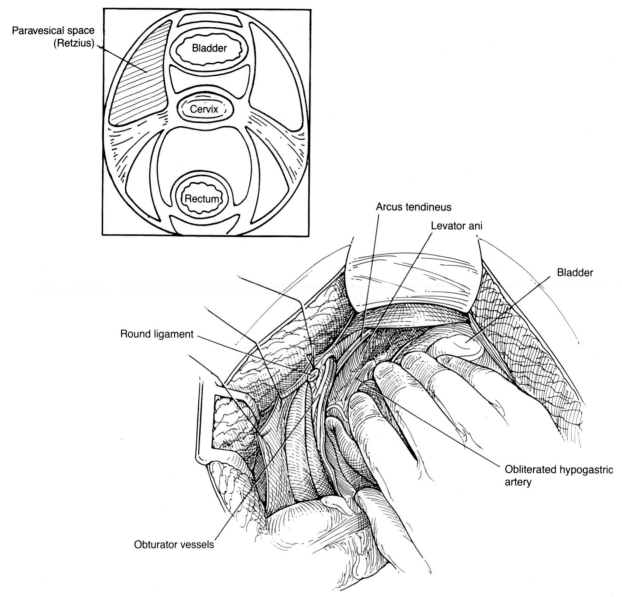

Figure 10–4. Laterally, the paravesical spaces are formed, exposing the obturator internus muscle, obturator vessels and nerve, levator ani, and frontal aspect of the cardinal ligament.

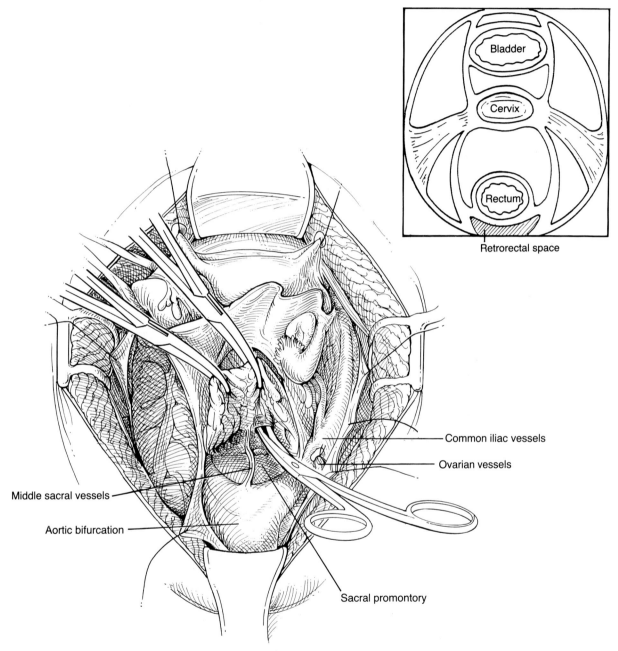

Bladder

Cervix

Rectum

Retrorectal space

Common iliac vessels

Ovarian vessels

Middle sacral vessels

Aortic bifurcation

Sacral promontory

Figure 10–5. Posteriorly, the retrorectal space is opened by separating anteriorly the rectum from the hollow of the sacrum and carrying the dissection down to the levator ani.

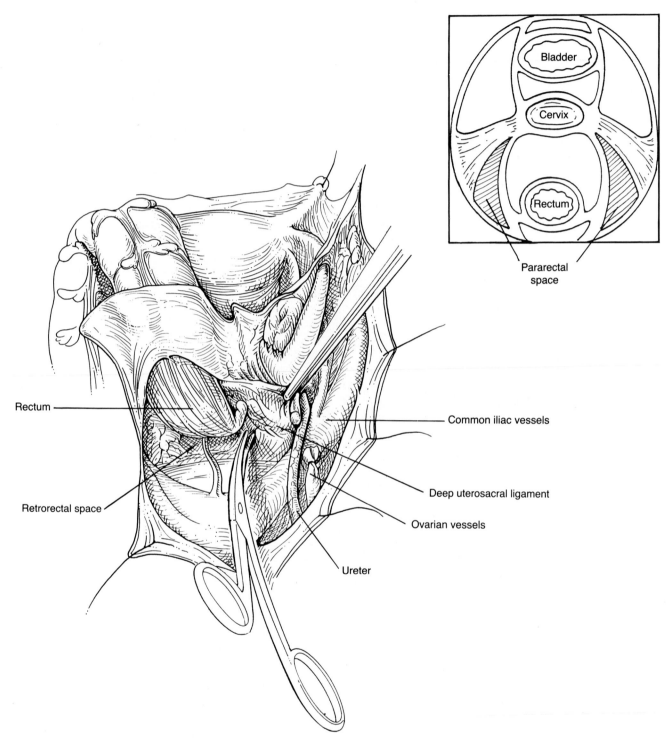

Bladder

Cervix

Rectum

Pararectal
space

Rectum

Retrorectal space

Common iliac vessels

Deep uterosacral ligament

Ovarian vessels

Ureter

Figure 10–6. Extending the dissection laterally and through the most posterior and inferior aspect of the uterosacral ligament, the pararectal fossa is entered and developed, exposing laterally the hypogastric vessels, anteriorly the dorsal aspect of the cardinal ligament, and superiorly and medially the ureter.

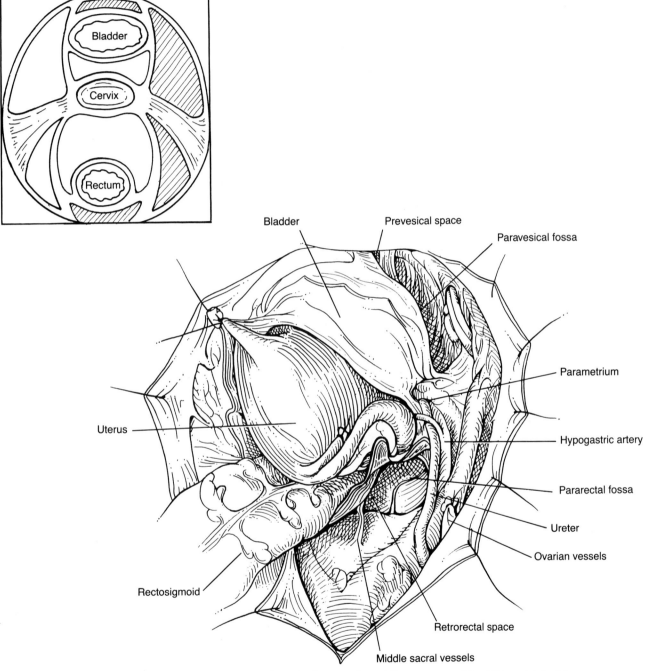

Figure 10–7. Complete mobilization of the pelvic structures by the creation of these spaces. It is at this point that the most lateral aspect of the parametrial structures can be biopsied to determine resectability.

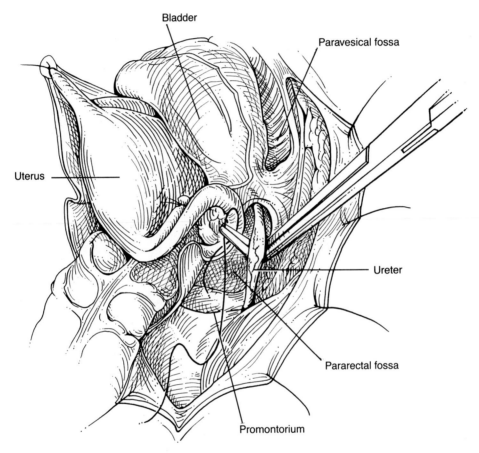

Figure 10–8. The ureters are isolated and cut just below the point of crossing the iliac vessels. They are catheterized with the catheter advanced to the renal pelvis and connected to plastic bags to ascertain urinary output during surgery.

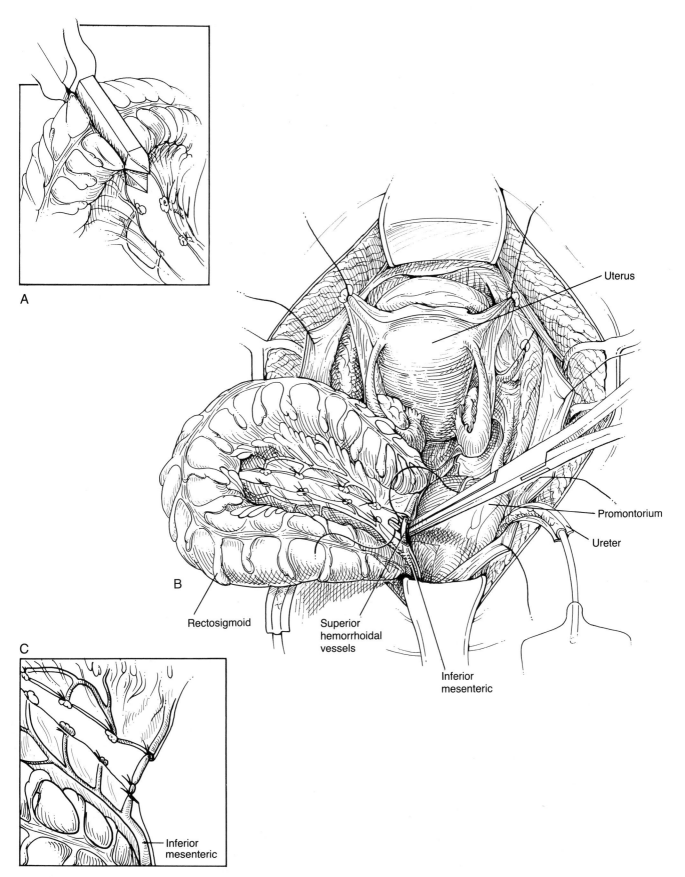

A

B

Rectosigmoid

Superior
hemorrhoidal
vessels

Inferior
mesenteric

Uterus

Promontorium

Ureter

C

Inferior
mesenteric

Figure 10–9. *A–C,* The sigmoid colon is sectioned with the gastrointestinal anastomosis (GIA) stapler. The sigmoid mesentery, including the superior hemorrhoidal vessels, is serially cut and ligated down to the retrorectal space. Sectioning of the sigmoid can be done before or after mesenteric vessels are cut. A more conservative resection of the sigmoid is performed if the sigmoid colon is to be used as a bladder substitute.

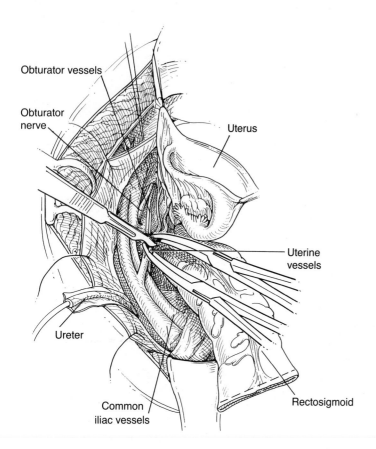

Figure 10–10. Lymphadenectomy is performed by dissecting the areolar tissue over the iliac vessels down to Poupart's ligament. The internal iliac vessels are exposed and ligated and cut. The distal end of the hypogastric artery is retracted downward and medially, exposing its branches, which are individually ligated and cut.

Figure 10–11. Ligation of the obturator vessels. The division of the hypogastric vein and tributaries must be done with extreme care because major blood loss can occur during this part of the operation. When tumor is predominantly central or in the anteroposterior plane, we have opted not to sacrifice the internal iliac vessels and carried the dissection just medial to them.

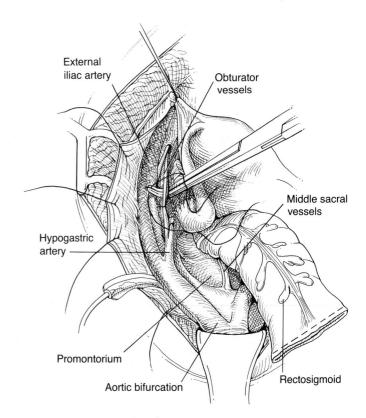

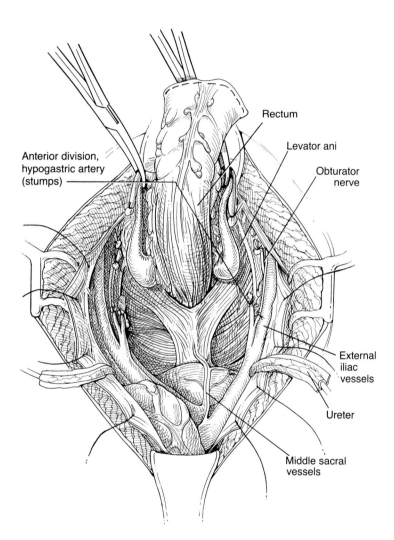

Anterior division,
hypogastric artery
(stumps)

Rectum

Levator ani

Obturator
nerve

External
iliac
vessels

Ureter

Middle sacral
vessels

Figure 10–12. All the attachments of the pelvic viscera have been sectioned down to the levator ani.

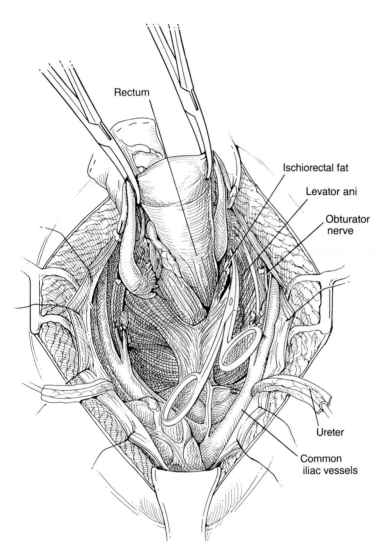

Rectum

Ischiorectal fat

Levator ani

Obturator nerve

Ureter

Common iliac vessels

Figure 10–13. If reconstruction of the vagina is not anticipated or if the cancer is confined to the upper half of the vagina, the operation is completed through the abdomen ``in toto.'' The levator ani is incised sharply, leaving a collar of muscle around the pelvic viscera, exposing the ischiorectal fossa.

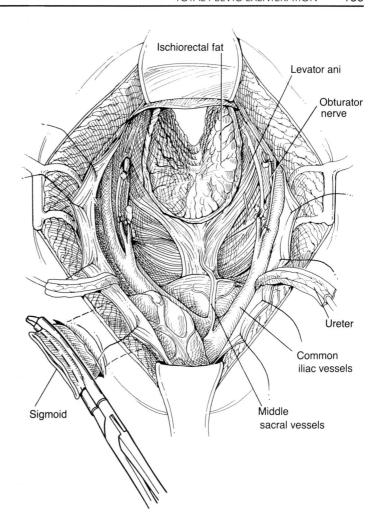

Ischiorectal fat

Levator ani

Obturator nerve

Ureter

Common iliac vessels

Middle sacral vessels

Sigmoid

Figure 10–14. The completed operation shown from above, with the perineal defect. The sigmoid colon has been pulled through a skin incision for later maturation.

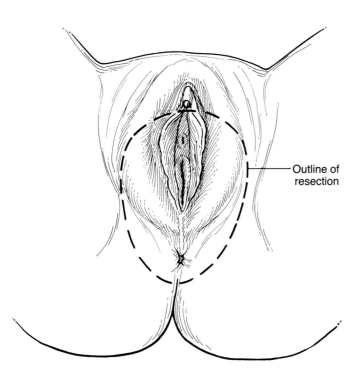

Outline of resection

Figure 10–15. The perineal phase of the operation is begun with an outline of the area of resection.

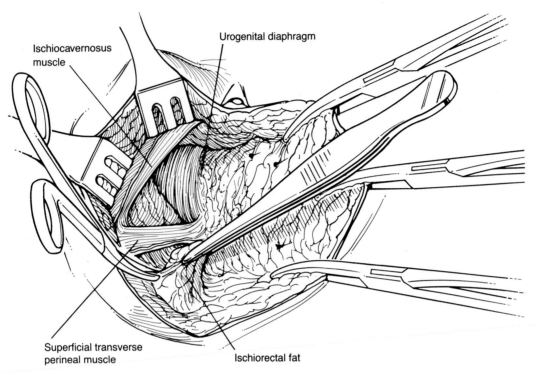

Figure 10–16. The incision is carried down to the fat of the ischiorectal fossa, exposing the superficial transverse perineal muscle and the ischiocavernosus.

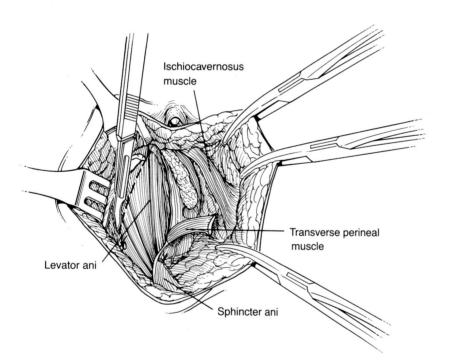

Figure 10–17. The superficial transverse perineal muscle is cut close to the ischial tuberosity. The levator ani is dissected and resected as far lateral as it is feasible.

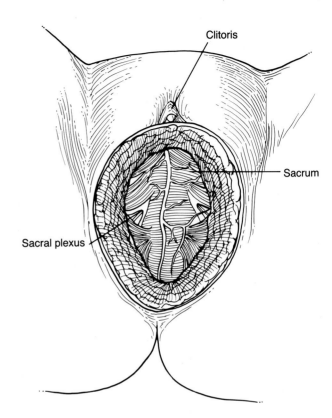

Figure 10–18. Guided by the assistant from the abdominal side, the specimen is removed through the perineal defect. Following removal, a pelvic lid, if feasible, may be created using peritoneum or omentum. If no reconstruction is performed, the empty pelvis is packed with gauze that is removed 5 to 7 days after surgery.

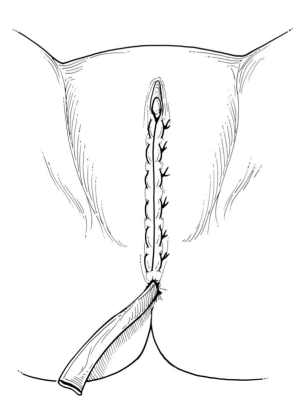

Figure 10–19. Alternately, the perineal defect is closed with drainage at the most dependent portion. For vaginal reconstruction, see Chapter 16.

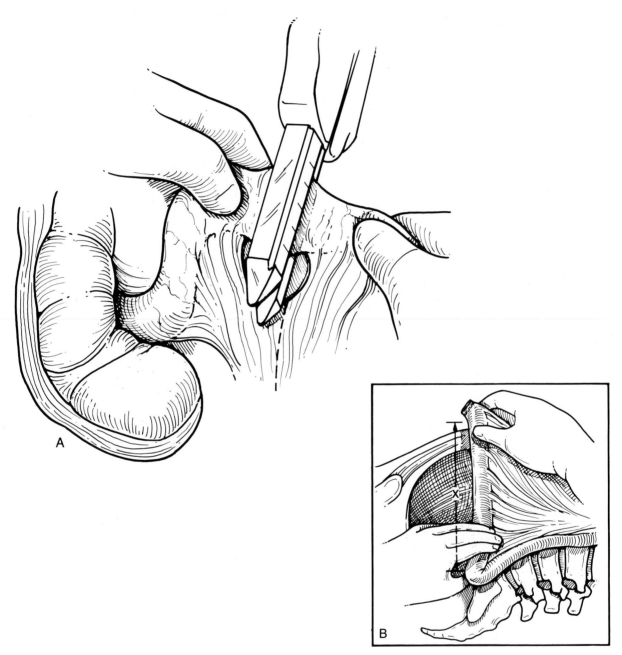

Figure 10–20. *A,* The ileal loop is isolated. Sigmoid or transverse colon conduits are alternatives. The distal segment is divided with the GI stapler as for a small bowel resection. The division should be at least 8 cm from the ileocecal valve. *B,* The length of the loop is determined by placing the distal end at the level of the stomal site and the proximal end at the level of the promontory, where it will be anchored.

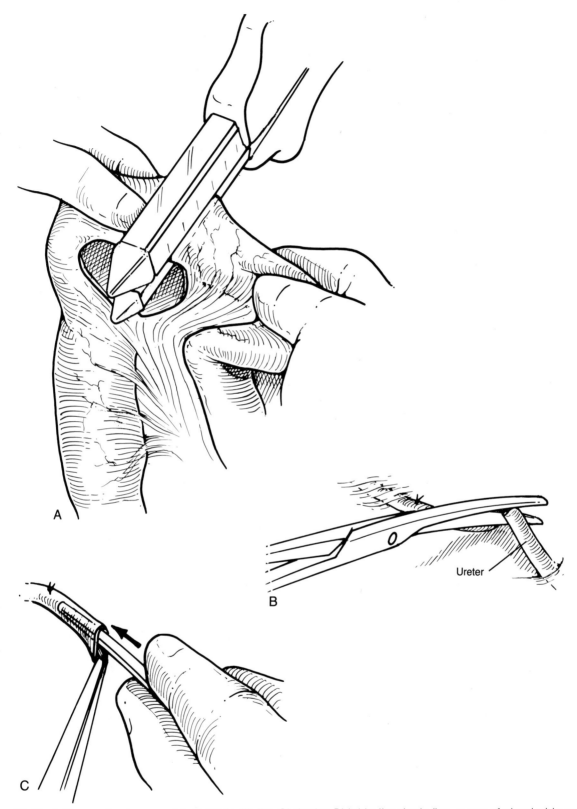

Figure 10–21. *A,* The proximal segment is divided with the GI stapler. Distal to the staple line, a row of absorbable material or absorbable staples (Polysorb) is placed to prevent formation of calculi that might occur if urine were in contact with the metal staples. The proximal or distal end of the loop is marked with a suture to help in identifying it during later steps of the operation. *B,* The ureter, if not already sectioned, is divided at the preselected level, and the anterior wall is marked with a suture to prevent twisting during the procedure. When possible, enough peritoneum is left attached to the ureter to preserve its blood supply and reinforce the uretero-intestinal anastomosis. *C,* If a ureteral catheter was not placed at the time of the original ureteral division, a 6 to 8 F single J catheter is threaded proximally to the renal pelvis.

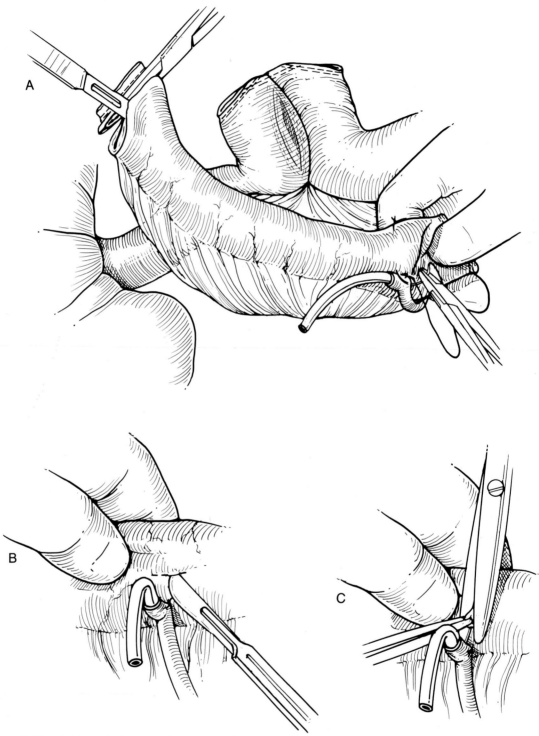

Figure 10–22. *A,* The distal staple line is excised. The ureter is anchored with three fine nonabsorbable sutures to the ileal loop (posterior outer layer of the anastomosis). *B,* The bowel seromuscular layer is opened transversely with a scalpel, causing the mucosa to protrude. *C,* A small button of mucosa is excised with Metzenbaum scissors.

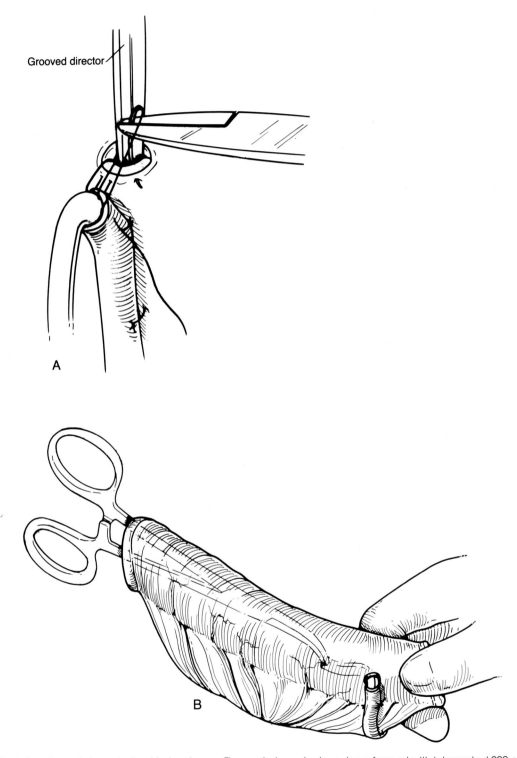

Figure 10–23. *A,* Anastomosis is carried out in two layers. The posterior outer layer is performed with interrupted 000 or 0000 sutures of nonabsorbable material. The posterior inner layer is performed by placing one medial and two angle sutures of 0000 absorbable material, taking care to keep the knots outside the bowel lumen. A grooved director is very useful in this step of the procedure. *B,* Using long curved forceps, the surgeon draws the ureteral catheter through the distal end of the loop.

Illustration continued on following page

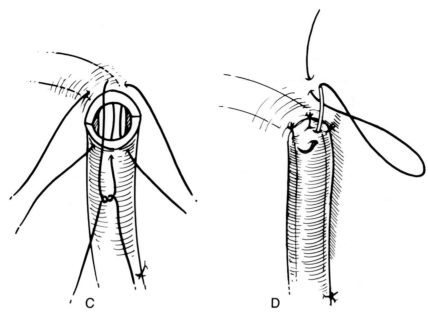

Figure 10-23 *Continued C,* The anterior inner layer is placed. *D,* The outer layer of anastomosis is performed, completing the anastomosis.

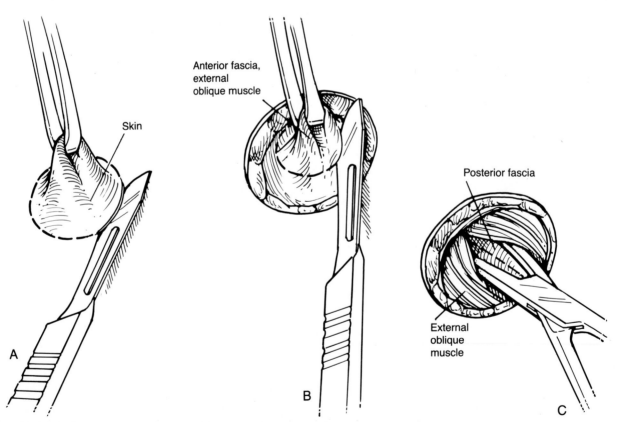

Figure 10-24. *A,* The stoma site is prepared by cutting away a small button of skin. *B,* After exposing the anterior fascia, the surgeon also removes a small button of this tissue. *C,* The muscle layer is separated and the posterior fascia and peritoneum incised.

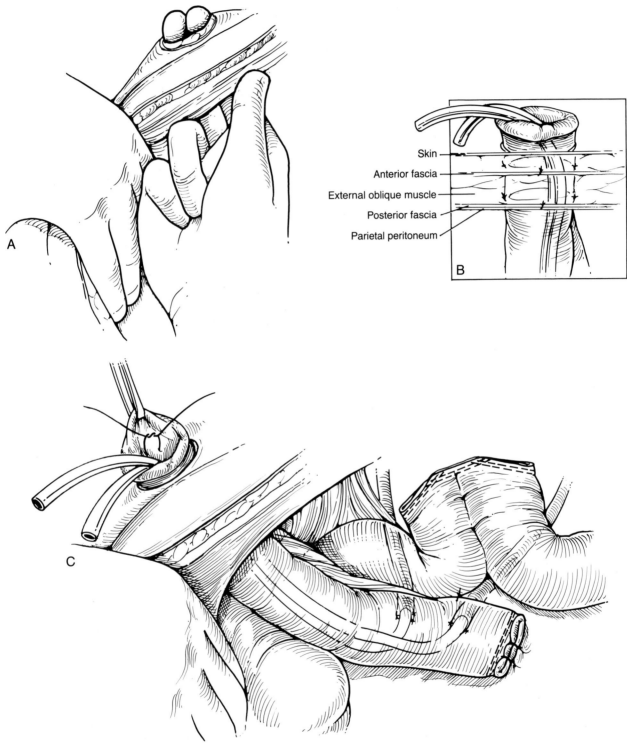

Skin
Anterior fascia
External oblique muscle
Posterior fascia
Parietal peritoneum

Figure 10–25. *A,* The stoma should be two fingers in width to prevent compromise of the blood supply of the loop. *B,* The loop is pulled through the stoma; four sutures of nonabsorbable material anchor the loop to the anterior fascia. A few interrupted sutures are placed between the parietal peritoneum and the loop to prevent peristomal hernias and to decrease tension at the stoma site. *C,* The ureteral splints are anchored to the mucosa of the loop to prevent accidental removal.

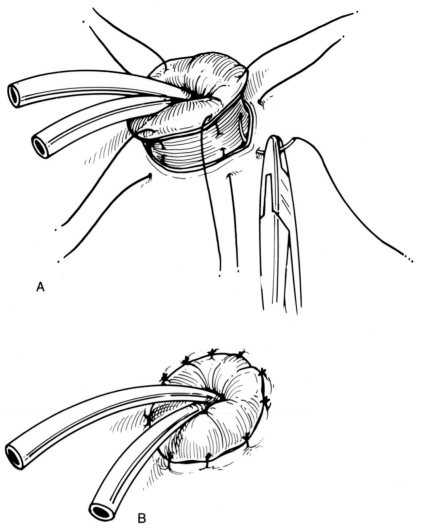

Figure 10–26. *A* and *B*, A rosebud stoma is fashioned with interrupted sutures of absorbable material. The suture passes through the seromuscular layer of skin and all layers of the bowel at its edge. The abdomen is closed in layers or alternatively by mass closure.

REFERENCES

1. Brunschwig A: Complete excision of pelvic viscera for advanced carcinoma. Cancer 1:177–183, 1948.
2. Symmonds RE, Pratt JH, and Webb MJ: Exenterative operations: Experience with 198 patients. Am J Obstet Gynecol 121:907–915, 1975.
3. Rutledge FN, Smith JP, Wharton JT, and O'Quinn AG: Pelvic exenteration: Analysis of 296 patients. Am J Obstet Gynecol 129:881–890, 1977.
4. Meigs JV, Brunschwig A: A proposed classification for cases of cancer of the cervix treated by surgery. Am J Obstet Gynecol 64:413–415, 1952.
5. Bricker EM, Butcher HR Jr, Lawler WH Jr, and McAfee CA: Surgical treatment of advanced and recurrent cancer of pelvic viscera: An evaluation of ten years' experience. Ann Surg 152:388–402, 1960.
6. Valle G, Ferraris G: Use of the omentum to contain the intestines in pelvic exenteration. Obstet Gynecol 110:696–701, 1971.
7. Morley GW, Lindenauer SM: Peritoneal graft in total pelvic exenteration. Am J Obstet Gynecol 110:696–701, 1971.
8. McCraw JB, Massey FM, Shanklin KD, and Horton CE: Vaginal reconstruction with gracilis myocutaneous flaps. Plast Reconstr Surg 58:176–183, 1976.

11

Anterior and Posterior Pelvic Exenteration

Mark J. Messing, M.D.

Total pelvic exenteration is an operation that has evolved extensively in gynecologic oncology. Since the original introduction by Brunschwig in 1948, the operation has become less morbid, and better patient selection has resulted in lower mortality and improved survival. New areas of development include formation of continent urinary conduits and reanastomosis of the intestinal tract. Selection of patients with small central recurrences may present the option of preserving the intact urinary or intestinal tract.

The role of a more limited exenterative procedure has its place in the patient with a small recurrence that is limited to the anterior or posterior pelvis. Attempting to leave the bladder or rectum intact requires that the tissue quality be sufficient to allow for safe dissection and satisfactory healing. Because the tissue is usually irradiated to tolerance doses, the risk of fistula formation and dysfunction of the preserved organ is high. Retention of the bladder after a posterior exenteration holds a very high risk for fistula formation or dysfunction.

Contraindications to a limited exenterative procedure include all the proscriptions to total pelvic exenteration. Pelvic sidewall disease, para-aortic lymph node involvement, and distant metastases are absolute contraindications. Hydroureter, nerve root pain, and lymphedema are relative contraindications that require negative results of frozen-section biopsies along the sidewall before the definitive operation is undertaken.

Treatment failure because of a less than ultraradical procedure is a major concern when an anterior or posterior exenteration is done. There is no apparent survival difference for these limited procedures in carefully selected patients when compared with total exenteration.[4, 7, 8] Candidates for anterior exenteration have a better prognosis when the tumor is less than 3 cm, more than 1 year out from primary treatment, and confined to the cervix.[2]

PATHOPHYSIOLOGIC POTENTIAL CHANGES

The limited roles of an anterior or posterior exenteration are for the removal of a central tumor that clearly does not involve either the rectum or bladder, respectively. Patient selection includes those with tumors that are smaller and displaced far enough away from the anterior or posterior vaginal wall to allow for sufficient margin. Anterior exenteration is the more common of the two procedures. Preserving the blood supply to the rectum is an important part of the procedure. Avoiding cases that involve extensive dissection of the rectovaginal septum can reduce the risk of fistula formation.[5]

Posterior exenteration is a less commonly performed procedure. The surgical separation of the anterior vagina and cervix from the bladder can be extremely difficult in the irradiated patient. The ureters and bladder base are exposed to extensive dissection and potential surgical injury. Radiation and surgery can produce devascularization, placing these structures at risk for fistula formation. Bladder dysfunction due to the endarteritis and fibrosis from radiation may be worsened by denervation from a radical procedure.

The extent of the perineal phase should be individualized. A smaller tumor that does not extend to the distal vagina may allow preservation of the levators, distal vagina, rectum, anus, or urethra, depending on whether exenteration modification is practical. Preservation of the levators reduces the risks of perineal hernia formation. It is hoped that preservation of perineal anatomy reduces the loss of sexual identity.

POTENTIAL PROBLEM AREAS

Surgical reconstruction of the pelvic organs is an important part of the rehabilitation of exenteration patients. The creation of a neovagina is important in the sexually active patient, regardless of age. In addition, our preference for a myocutaneous flap reconstruction of the vagina provides soft tissue bulk to fill the pelvis and prevent bowel adherence to the raw peritoneal surfaces. Bowel obstruction has been shown to be the most common complication following pelvic exenteration.[4, 5] The flap allows nonirradiated tissue to bring additional blood supply to the pelvis, which, it is hoped, will reduce the risk of fistula formation. Myocutaneous flaps that have been used include unilateral or bilateral gracilis, bulbocavernosus, or unilateral rectus abdominis flaps. Ligation of the hypogastric artery should be avoided if one contemplates a myocutaneous flap based on one of the branches of this vessel.

Reconstructive procedures of the rectum can be performed in a supralevator procedure if sufficient rectum is available for reanastomosis. Stapling instruments greatly facilitate the reanastomotic procedure. A minimum of 6 cm of remaining rectum has been shown to result in improved healing in association with an omental wrap.[2] Mobilization of the omentum based on a left gastro-epiploic vessel allows for this excellent source of bulky soft tissue and blood supply to be used as a wrap around the anastomotic line. It also helps fill the pelvic defect.

Urinary tract reconstruction involves formation of a bowel segment conduit anastomosed to the ureters and brought through the abdominal wall. If the right colon and terminal ileum are in sufficiently good condition, a continent urinary pouch can be created using the Indiana or Miami method.[3, 6] In other cases, we prefer to use the transverse colon as an incontinent conduit because it is out of the radiation field, has a consistent blood supply, and is easily mobilized to the ureteral stumps.

ANTERIOR EXENTERATION

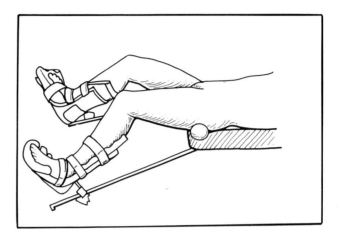

Figure 11–1. The patient is in a modified lithotomy position using the Allen stirrups. The thighs and knees are slightly flexed and the legs are abducted. This allows for adequate exposure to the perineum for a two-team approach.

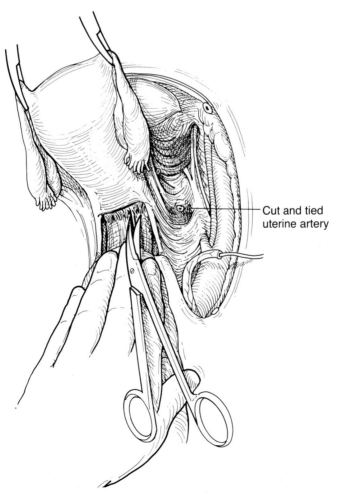

Cut and tied uterine artery

Figure 11–2. After opening the abdomen and exposing the pelvis, the lateral peritoneum is opened and the pelvic spaces are developed. The ureters have been divided at the pelvic brim. The uterine artery has been divided at its origin from the hypogastric artery. Upward traction on the sigmoid exposes the cul-de-sac and enhances dissection of the rectovaginal septum.

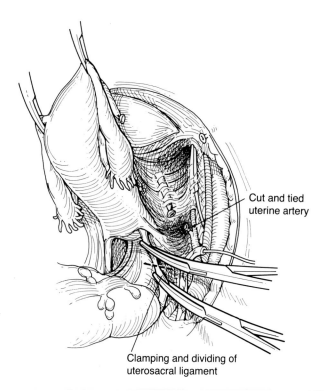

Cut and tied
uterine artery

Clamping and dividing of
uterosacral ligament

Figure 11-3. The uterosacral ligaments are divided close to their insertion.

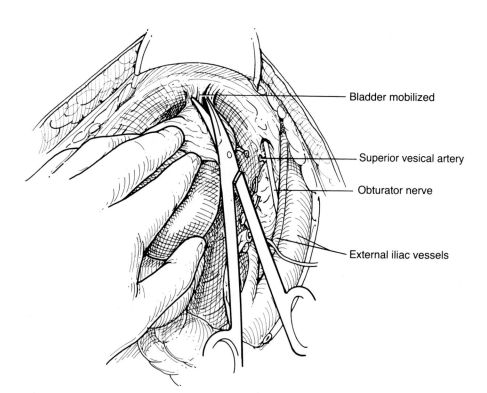

Bladder mobilized

Superior vesical artery

Obturator nerve

External iliac vessels

Figure 11-4. The anterior peritoneum is opened, and the space of Retzius is sharply developed. The bladder is fully mobilized from its attachments to the symphysis and the pelvic floor.

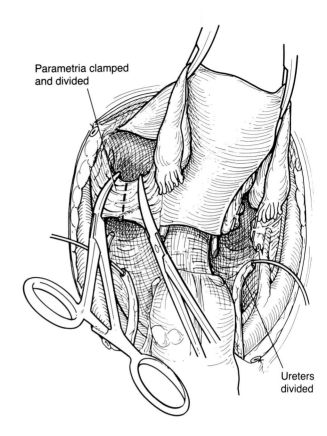

Parametria clamped
and divided

Ureters
divided

Figure 11–5. The cardinal ligaments are divided at the side-wall. The distal hypogastric artery is also divided during this step.

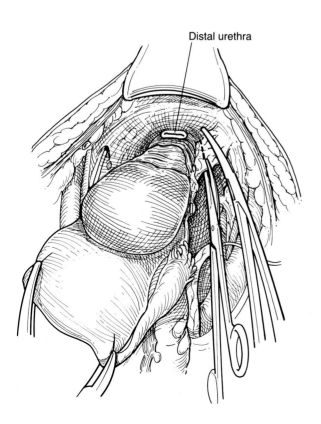

Distal urethra

Figure 11–6. Paravaginal attachments to the pelvic sidewall are divided down to the levators. The distal urethra above the pelvic diaphragm has been divided.

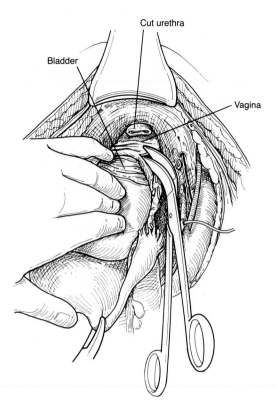

Figure 11–7. The vagina is divided and the specimen is removed.

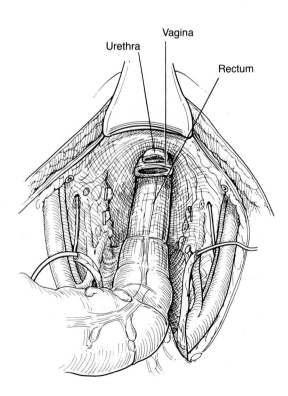

Figure 11–8. The field of dissection is shown, demonstrating the denuded rectum and exposed pelvic floor.

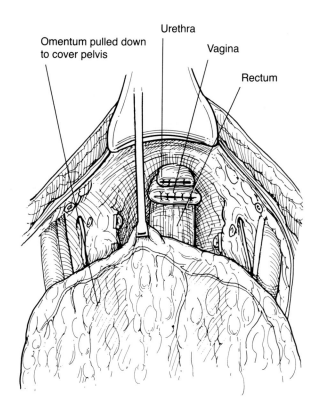

Figure 11–9. The remaining vagina and urethra are oversewn. The omentum has been mobilized and is brought down into the pelvis as a covering. The omentum is sutured to the psoas muscles and along the symphysis pubis.

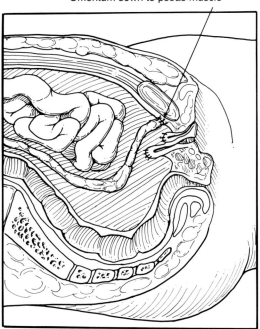

Figure 11–10. A lateral view of the pelvis shows how the omentum acts like a sling to prevent the bowel from falling into the pelvis.

TRANSVERSE COLON CONDUIT

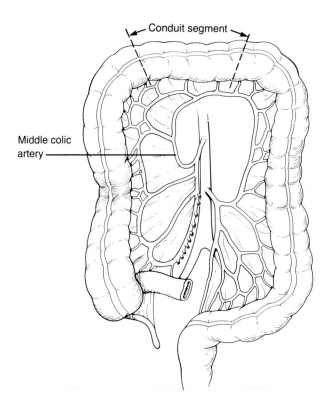

Figure 11–11. The transverse colon conduit is based on the blood supply of the middle colic artery. The omentum is mobilized off the transverse colon, exposing the lesser sac. The middle colic artery is palpated and transilluminated to identify a 15 to 20 cm segment supplied by the artery for the conduit.

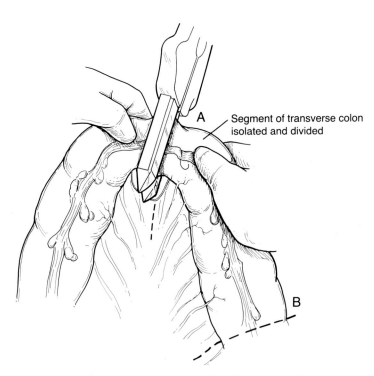

Figure 11–12. A gastrointestinal stapler is shown dividing one end (A) of the selected bowel segment. The opposite end of the segment (B) is also divided by the stapler.

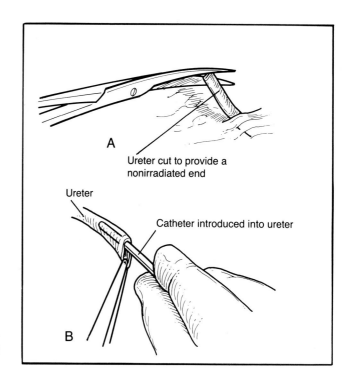

Figure 11–13. The ureter is freshly cut to provide a nonirradiated end for the anastomosis (*A*). A 7 Fr pediatric feeding tube or a single J ureteral catheter is used as a stent (*B*).

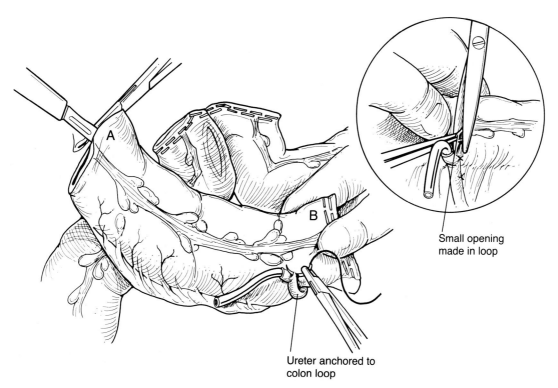

Figure 11–14. The proximal and distal transverse colon is reanastomosed using gastrointestinal staplers. The distal or proximal conduit end is opened, and the segment is irrigated to remove residual fecal material. The serosa of the ureter is sutured to the intestinal wall to stabilize the anastomotic line. *Insert,* A small opening is made into the colon segment along one of the tinea for the anastomosis.

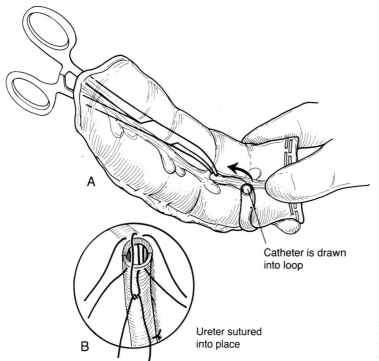

A

Catheter is drawn
into loop

B

Ureter sutured
into place

Figure 11–15. *A*, The stent is pulled into the conduit segment from the distal end. *B*, The ureter is sutured to the intestine segment utilizing 4–0 absorbable sutures. The anastomosis must include full thickness of both intestinal wall and ureter, applying mucosa to mucosa.

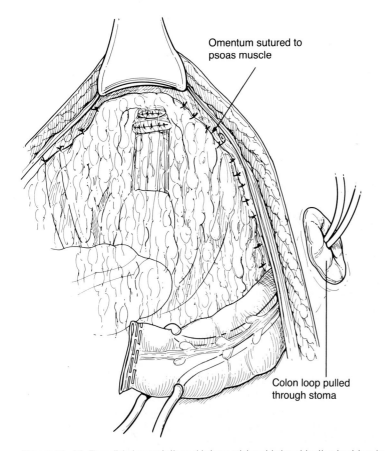

Omentum sutured to
psoas muscle

Colon loop pulled
through stoma

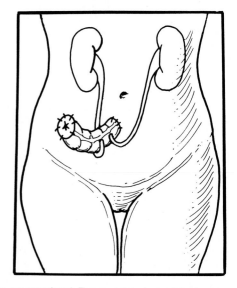

Figure 11–16. The distal conduit end is brought out lateral to the incision in the right lower quadrant. The quadrant can be chosen depending on conduit length and mobility. The proximal conduit end is sutured to the posterior peritoneum.

POSTERIOR EXENTERATION

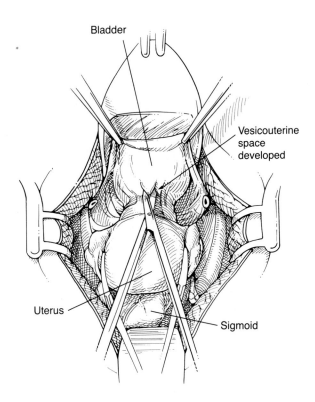

Figure 11-17. The abdomen has been opened and the pelvic structures exposed. The pelvic peritoneum has been opened and the pelvic spaces have been developed. The vesicouterine peritoneum is divided and the bladder is sharply mobilized off the cervix.

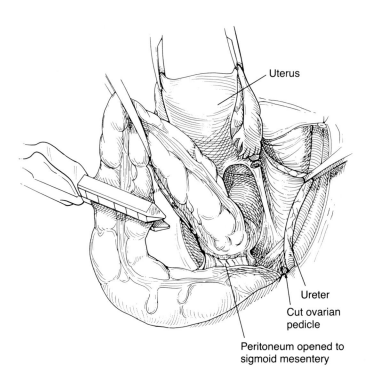

Figure 11-18. The sigmoid colon mesentery is divided and the sigmoid colon is divided at the pelvic brim.

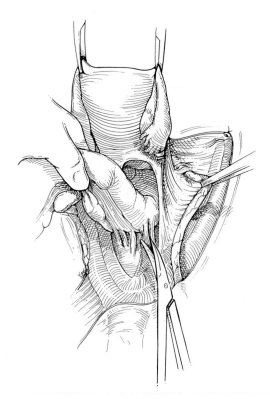

Figure 11-19. The presacral space is sharply developed.

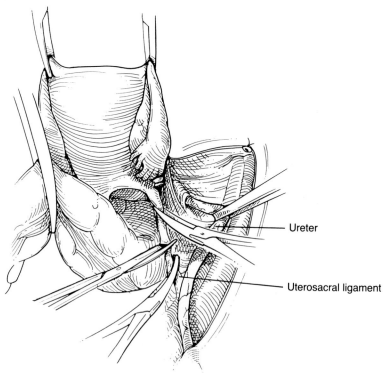

Ureter

Uterosacral ligament

Figure 11-20. The uterosacral ligaments are divided at their insertion.

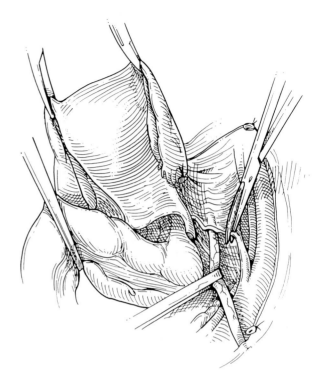

Figure 11-21. The uterine artery is ligated and divided at its origin from the hypogastric artery.

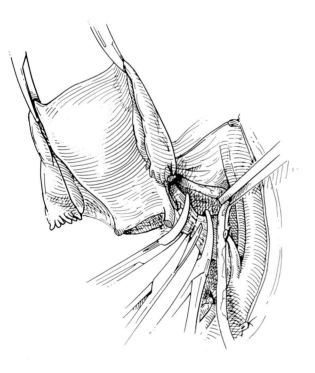

Figure 11-22. The ureter is mobilized from the cardinal ligament and retracted laterally. The cardinal ligaments are divided at the pelvic sidewall.

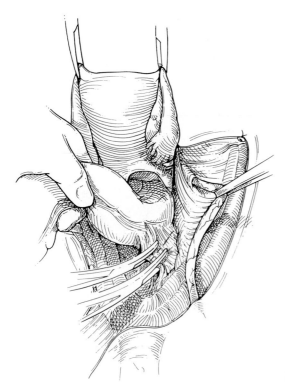

Figure 11-23. The rectal pillars are divided at the pelvic sidewall.

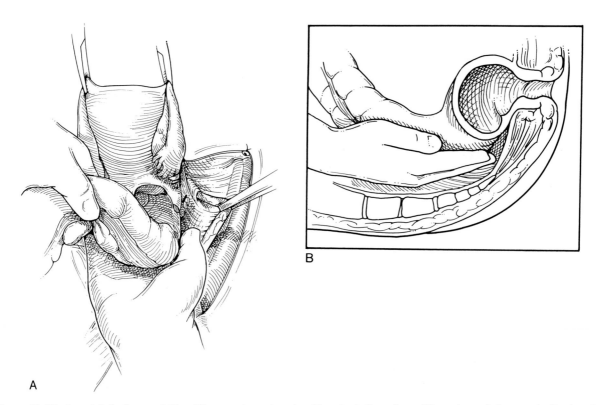

A

B

Figure 11-24. *A* and *B,* Further mobility of the specimen is gained by blunt dissection of the retrorectal space to the levators.

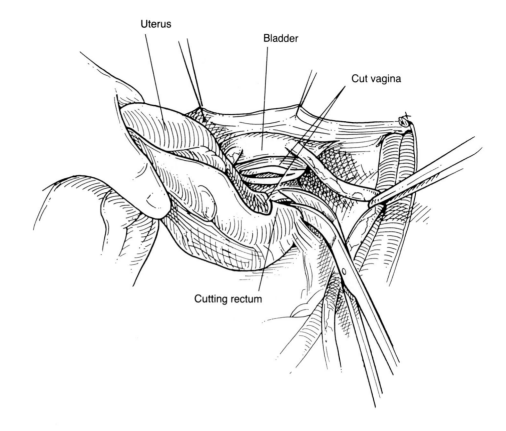

Uterus

Bladder

Cut vagina

Cutting rectum

Figure 11–25. In a supralevator exenteration, the specimen is divided at the level of the levator muscles.

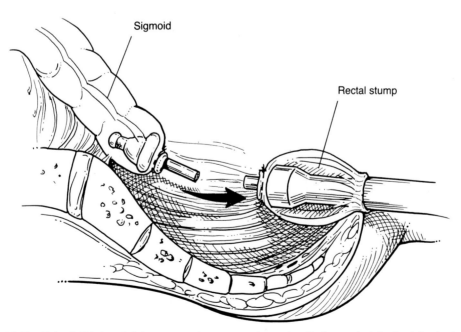

Sigmoid

Rectal stump

Figure 11–26. If sufficient distal rectal stump remains, an anastomosis with the gastrointestinal stapler is performed.

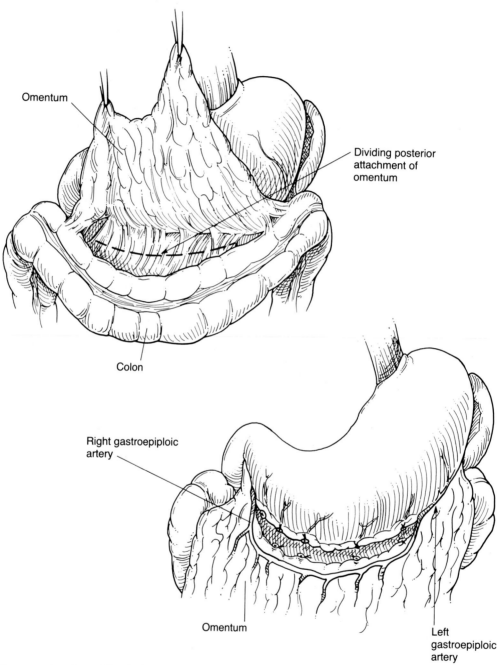

Figure 11–27. The omentum is mobilized off the transverse colon and the stomach. A pedicle graft is created based on the left gastroepiploic vessels.

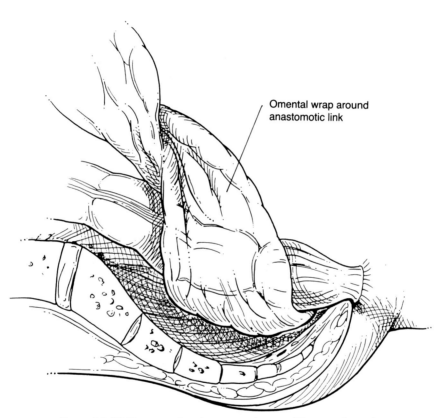

Omental wrap around
anastomotic link

Figure 11–28. The omentum is wrapped around the anastomosis.

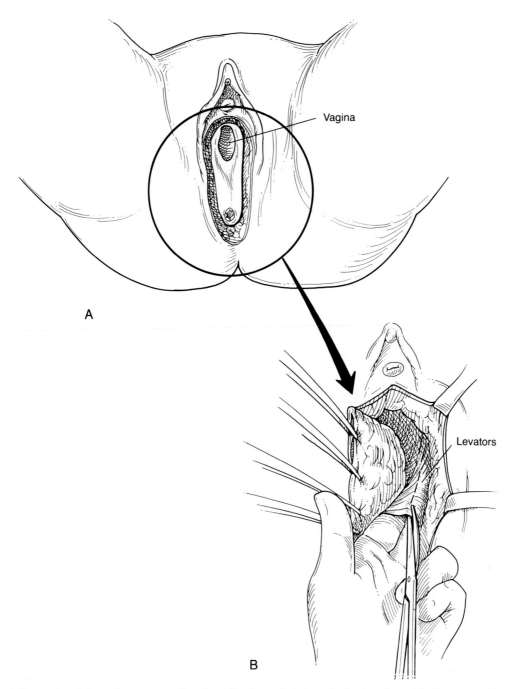

Figure 11–29. *A*, If a perineal phase is necessary, the dissection is carried down to the levators while the second team begins. The rectum is sutured closed and the dissection proceeds cephalad. *B*, The levators are divided from below with assistance from above.

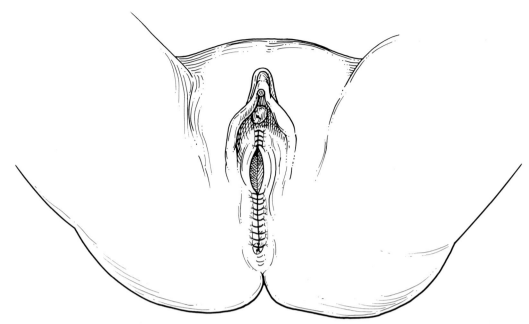

Figure 11–30. The completed operation may now proceed to a vaginal reconstruction if planned. The omentum is mobilized and used to create a pelvic lid to prevent intestines from adhering to the denuded pelvic floor. An end sigmoid colostomy is formed.

REFERENCES

1. Brunschwig A: Complete excision of pelvic viscera for advanced carcinoma. Cancer 1:177–183, 1948.
2. Hatch KD, Gelder MS, Soong S, et al: Pelvic exenteration with low rectal anastomosis: Survival, complications, and prognostic factors. Gynecol Oncol 38:462–467, 1990.
3. Mannel RS, Braly PS, Buller RE: Indiana pouch continent urinary reservoir in patients with previous pelvic irradiation. Obstet Gynecol 75:891–893, 1990.
4. Morley GW, Hopkins MP, Lindenauer SM, Roberts JA. Pelvic exenteration, University of Michigan: 100 patients at 5 years. Obstet Gynecol 74:934–943, 1989.
5. Orr JW, Shingleton HM, Hatch KD, et al: Gastrointestinal complications associated with pelvic exenteration. Am J Obstet Gynecol 145:325–332, 1983.
6. Penalver MA, Bejany DE, Averette HE, et al: Continent urinary diversion in gynecologic oncology. Gynecol Oncol 34:274–288, 1989.
7. Shingleton HM, Soong SJ, Gelder MS, et al: Clinical and histopathologic factors predicting recurrence and survival after pelvic exenteration for cancer of the cervix. Obstet Gynecol 73:1027–1034, 1989.
8. Symmonds RE, Pratt JH, Webb MJ: Exenterative operations: Experience with 198 patients. Am J Obstet Gynecol 121:907–918, 1975.

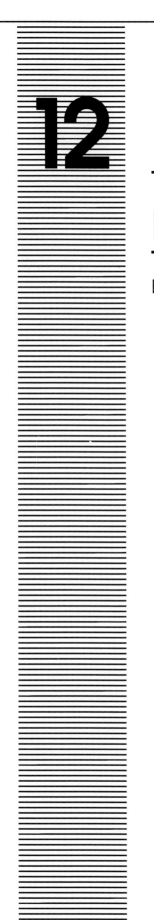

12

The Continent Urinary Reservoir

Laurel A. King, M.D.

The concept of continent urinary diversion is not new. In 1852, Simon performed the first ureterosigmoidostomy on a patient with congenital bladder exstrophy.[1] During the next 90 years, ureterosigmoidostomy with several modifications was the urinary diversion procedure of choice, although many attempts were made at utilizing isolated segments of the right colon for continent urinary diversion. In 1950, Gilchrist published a series of 12 cases in which a right colon diversion was used.[2] Almost simultaneously, Bricker popularized the idea of an ileal conduit.[3] The ease of construction and rapidity of forming the ileal conduit, plus the lack of acceptance by patients to perform self-catheterization, made the ileal conduit the urinary diversion procedure of choice from 1950 to 1970.

The modern era of continent urinary diversion came about for two reasons: (1) the gradual acceptance by physicians of the concept of clean, intermittent self-catheterization by patients; and (2) the adaptation of the Kock continent ileostomy as a urinary reservoir.[4, 5] Shortly after the acceptance of the Kock pouch, work began anew on the use of the right colon segment for continent diversion.

The procedure that will be described is our modification of the continent urinary pouches developed by Penalver and colleagues at the University of Miami[6] and the Indiana pouch developed by Rowland and associates at Indiana University.[7]

Indications for continent urinary diversions in women with gynecologic malignancies are: (1) for patients who are undergoing exenterative procedures for treatment of primary or recurrent gynecologic malignancies; and (2) for treatment of complications of cancer therapy, specifically unrepairable vesicovaginal fistulas. Patients should have a strong motivation to retain a normal body image and must understand and be willing to perform self-catheterization on a frequent basis for the remainder of their lives. Patients also must be physically able to catheterize and be mentally fit. Poor candidates for continent urinary diversion include those with crippling arthritis or those psychologically unable to tolerate the catheterization of the pouch at frequent intervals.

The ideal urinary diversion has not yet been developed. However, many years of experience with ileal and colon conduits have indicated that the vast majority of these patients undergo upper tract deterioration after 3 to 5 years of conduit existence. It is hoped that the use of low-pressure continent urinary reservoirs will lessen the chance of upper tract deterioration and allow preservation of a more natural body habitus for women who already have physical and psychological stigmata of genital tract cancer.

PREOPERATIVE PATIENT PREPARATION

The patient should have a mechanical and antibiotic bowel preparation prior to pouch formation. This can be accomplished by whatever mechanical method (e.g., GoLytely) is favored by the operating surgeon. Oral antibiotics should also be administered as well as prophylactic intravenous antibiotics. It is important to ensure that a thorough mechanical bowel preparation is accomplished so that when the electrocautery is used to open the bowel, there is no explosion secondary to bowel gas.

The enterostomal therapist should see the patient prior to the proposed surgical procedure, thus facilitating selection of an appropriate site for the ileal stoma placement. However, this is not a hard and fast rule, because it is critical to place the ileal stoma on the abdominal wall where it is at a 90-degree angle to the pouch and ileocecal valve, facilitating catheterization by the patient. It should be noted that the ileal stoma can be placed anywhere on the abdominal wall (i.e., right lower quadrant in the hairline or out through the umbilicus). Additional considerations for placement of the ileal stoma site would be necessary if additional reconstructive procedures (i.e., rectus flaps, colostomy) are planned. This procedure is not technically demanding, but it does take longer than an ileal or colon conduit, and strict attention to detail is necessary during pouch construction.

POTENTIAL PROBLEM AREAS

Patients who have significant radiation damage to the ileocecal segment are not candidates for this type of continent urinary diversion. If continent diversion is desired, a Kock-type urinary pouch would be necessary. Another possible problem area is in patients who have had a previous cholecystectomy. The colon must be mobilized from the right hepatic flexure, and significant bleeding can ensue if dense adhesions are present.

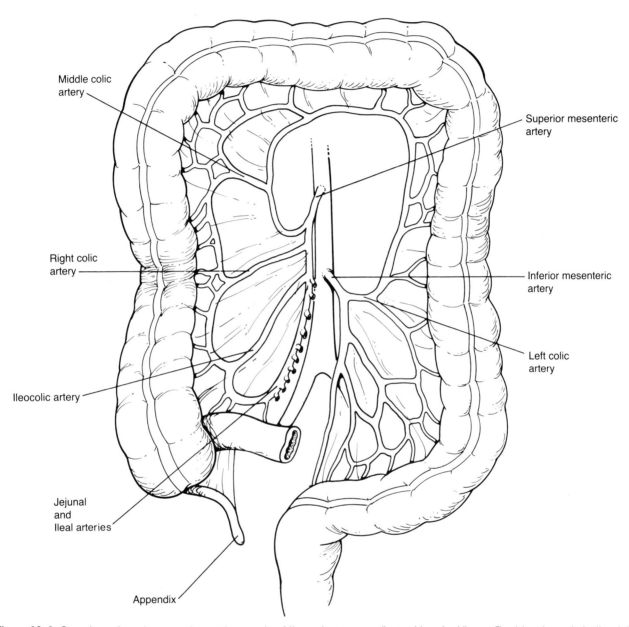

Figure 12-1. Overview of anatomy and vascular supply of the colon, appendix, and terminal ileum. The blood supply to the right colon and terminal ileum arises from the superior mesenteric artery. Specifically, a rich blood supply to the right colon is provided by the middle colic artery, right colic artery, and ileocolic artery.

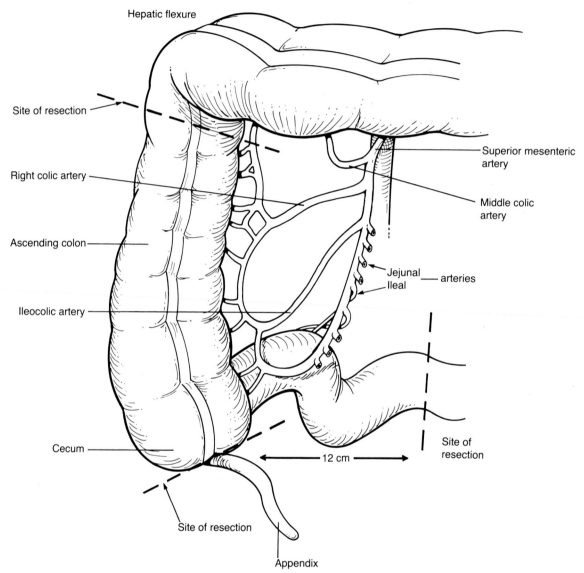

Figure 12-2. The anatomic location and vascularity of the right colon segment utilized for formation of the continent urinary pouch. Illustrated are the anatomic sites of division for creation of the continent pouch. The ascending colon is divided distal to the right colic artery. The terminal ileum is divided approximately 12 cm from the ileocecal valve. The resection can be accomplished with the use of surgical staplers or by intestinal clamps. If the appendix is present, it should be removed. The ileocecal segment has a rich blood supply derived from the right colic artery and the ileocolic artery. If one is performing the Miami pouch type of urinary diversion, the transverse colon would be divided distal to the middle colic artery.

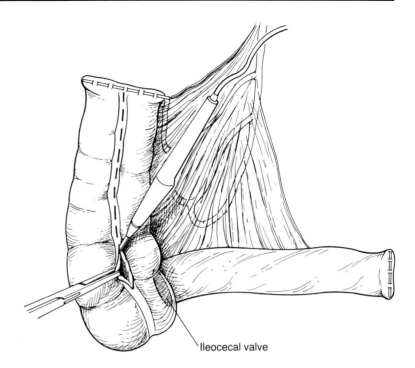

Figure 12–3. The prepared intestinal segment is now ready for detubularization. Using the electrocautery, one opens the colon approximately 1½ inches cephalad to the ileocecal valve along the tenia.

Ileocecal valve

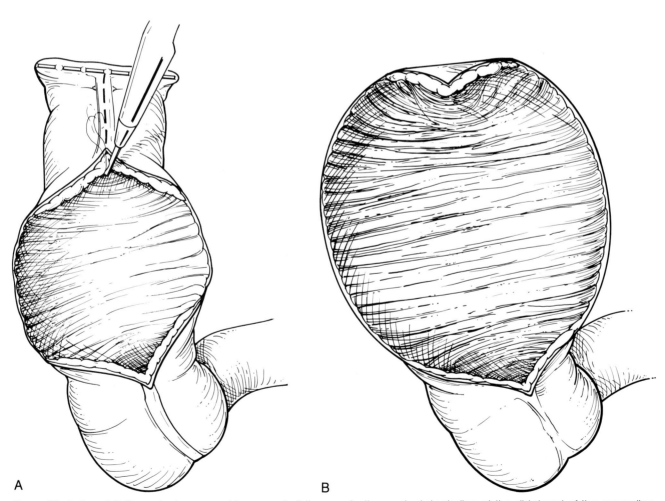

A

B

Figure 12–4. *A* and *B,* The colonic segment is opened all the way to the surgical staple line at the distal end of the ascending colon.

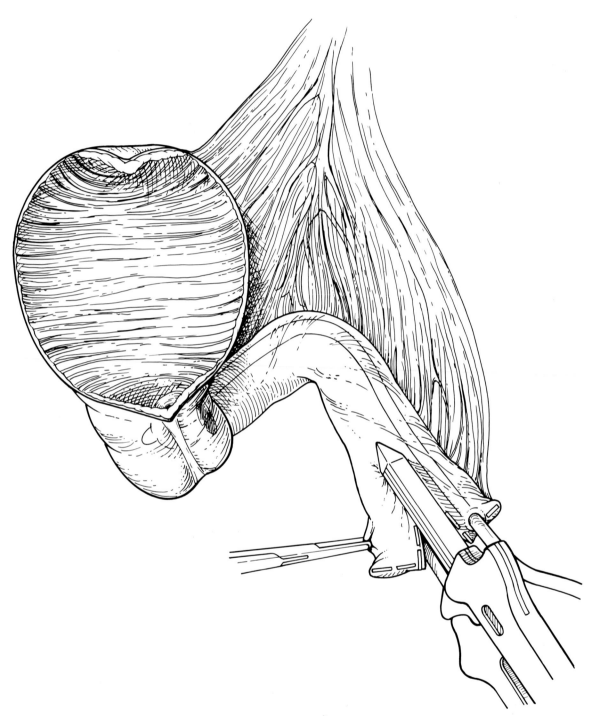

Figure 12–5. The continent mechanism is created in two parts. First, the terminal ileal segment is tapered down over a 14 French Foley catheter. This can be accomplished using an intestinal dividing and stapling device such as a GIA 80 or, in the Indiana pouch, imbricating sutures.

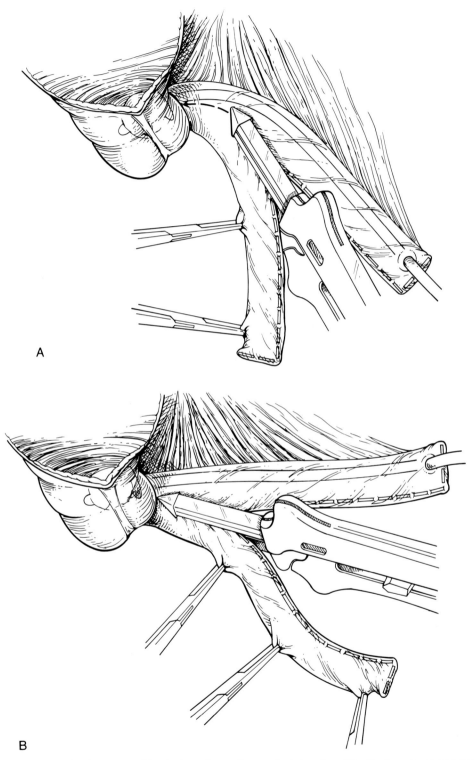

A

B

Figure 12-6. *A* and *B,* The tapering is accomplished along the antimesenteric border of the ileal segment. The entire ileal segment is tapered to the diameter of the 14 French catheter (down to the ileocecal valve). The excess ileum is trimmed away, leaving the tapered segment.

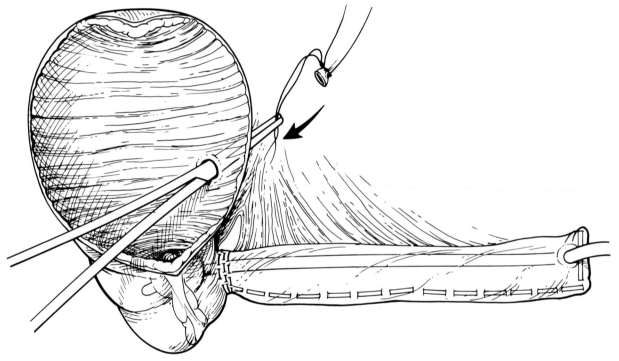

Figure 12–7. The second part of the continent mechanism is accomplished by plication of the ileocecal valve. The area of the ileocecal valve is plicated using concentric purse-string sutures of 0 silk or polypropylene. If a hole is made in an avascular portion of the ileal mesentery at the area of the ileocecal valve, passage of the needle and suture material is facilitated during purse-string suturing. The sutures are placed, but not tied, until all sutures are placed. They are tied down snugly, but not tight enough to strangulate the ileocecal valve. Thus, pressures in the ileal segment and the ileal valve are increased, and the formation of the continent mechanism is completed. The left ureter shown is being brought into the colon segment.

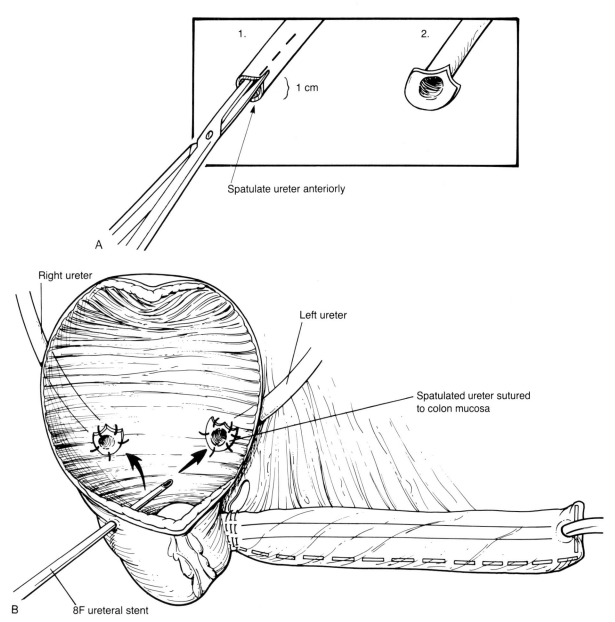

Figure 12–8. *A* and *B,* Prior to beginning the continent diversion, the ureters have been transected (usually at the pelvic brim) and mobilized so that they are able to be brought to the area where the continent pouch will be located without tension. If necessary, the left ureter can be brought through or under the mesentery of the colon to facilitate its placement into the urinary pouch. An appropriate site is selected on what will be the posterior wall of the pouch, and a long thin clamp is used to perforate the colon and pull the ureter through. An approximately 1-cm segment of ureter is brought into the pouch. For ease of ureterointestinal anastomosis, the ureter should be secured posteriorly to the pouch by suturing the adventitial tissue of the ureter to the seromuscular layers of the pouch with three or four permanent 3-0 sutures. The ureter is spatulated to increase the lumen diameter. The ureter is sutured directly to the colon and is not tunneled. We use 4-0 polyglycolic suture. This is a full-thickness approximation of the colon and ureter. Once both ureters have been sutured into the pouch, two #8 French ureterointestinal stents or long pediatric feeding tubes are placed retrograde into the renal pelvis. If a feeding tube is used, it should be sutured to the ureter with 4-0 chromic to ensure against displacement due to ureteral peristalsis.

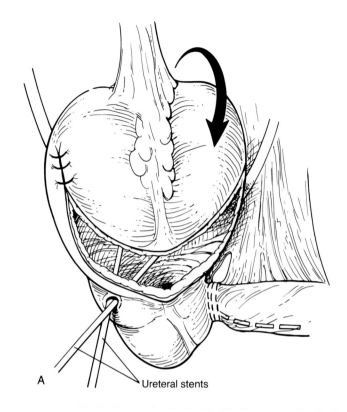

Ureteral stents

A

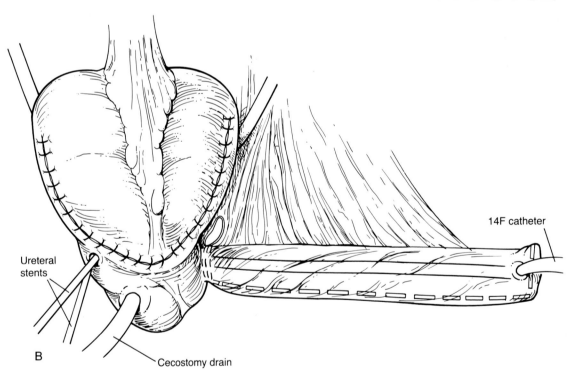

Ureteral
stents

14F catheter

B

Cecostomy drain

Figure 12–9. *A* and *B,* The colon is reconfigured using the Heineke-Mikulicz reconfiguration, which involves folding the detubular- ized colon segment caudad. A 24 French "mushroom" drain is placed through the anterior pouch wall to effect drainage and is secured to the skin with a purse-string suture. (This is optional.) The ureterointestinal stents (or feeding tubes) are also brought out anteriorly through the pouch and secured with purse-string sutures. The new anterior wall of the pouch is then sutured with a single-layer closure. Alternatively, the pouch can be stapled with absorbable polyglycolic acid staples. If the absorbable staples are used, the areas between the staple lines should be sutured to effect a water-tight closure.

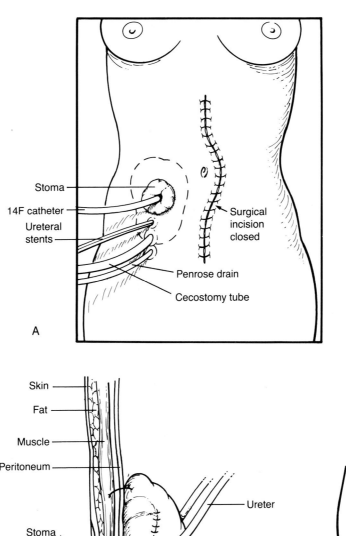

Stoma

14F catheter

Ureteral
stents

Surgical
incision
closed

Penrose drain

Cecostomy tube

A

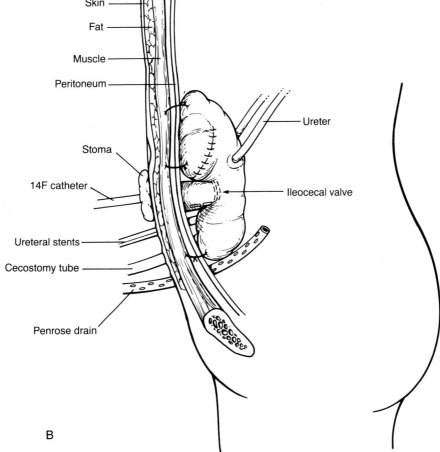

Skin

Fat

Muscle

Peritoneum

Ureter

Stoma

14F catheter

Ileocecal valve

Ureteral stents

Cecostomy tube

Penrose drain

B

Figure 12–10. *A* and *B,* The site for the ileal stoma is selected on the anterior abdominal wall and then incised through all abdominal tissue layers. The stoma is created for catheterization and the 14 French catheter should exit the pouch through this stoma. It is critical that the ileal segment be at a 90-degree angle with the abdominal wall so that catheterization is a ``straight shot.'' The pouch may be sutured to the abdominal wall to accomplish this. All stents and drainage tubes are brought out the anterior abdominal wall and secured. The pouch may also be anchored posteriorly (i.e., to the sacrum).

CONCLUDING MANAGEMENT COMMENTS

If desired, the pouch can be filled with sterile milk, indigo carmine, or methylene blue solution to check for leaks. Small leaks do not have to be sutured, especially in the area of the ureterointestinal anastomosis, because these should heal with appropriate drainage.

A Penrose or sump drain should be seated behind the pouch in the area of the ureterointestinal anastomosis to effect drainage in case there is a urinary leak. The cecostomy drain (optional) and ureteral stents are brought up through separate abdominal incisions and secured. Alternatively, the ureteral stents could be brought out with the 14 French catheter via the tapered ileal segment.

Once the abdominal incision is closed, the ileal segment can be fashioned into a stoma. The stoma is secured to the skin in the usual "rosebud" manner using 3-0 polyglycolic acid suture. The ileal segment should be brought up through the abdominal wall in as straight a manner as possible so that there is a "straight shot" for catheterization into the pouch, aiding the patient in later catheterization of the pouch. One can also secure the pouch anteriorly to the abdominal wall with 3-0 permanent or absorbable sutures to ensure fixation.

Irrigation of the pouch with 30 to 60 ml of saline should begin on the first postoperative day. It is necessary to irrigate the pouch every 4 to 8 hours through the cecostomy or 14 French catheter to remove intestinal mucus. Mucus production usually decreases, but it may be necessary for the patient to irrigate out mucus after her discharge from the hospital.

Two weeks post procedures, a pouch-o-gram and intravenous pyelography (IVP) are done to check for leaks. If no leaks are present, the ureteral stents may be removed. The patient can then initiate catheterization—initially at 2-hour intervals and later increased to 4- to 5-hour intervals. Once the patient can catheterize the pouch successfully, she can be discharged. Once she is comfortable using self-catheterization, the cecostomy drain (if placed) can be removed.

REFERENCES

1. Simon J: Ectopia vesical (absence of the anterior walls of the bladder and pubic abdominal parietes); operation for directing orifices of the ureters in the rectum; temporary success; subsequent death; autopsy. Lancet 2:568; 1852.
2. Gilchrist RF, Merricks JW, Hamlin HH, Rieger IT: Construction of a substitute bladder and urethra. Surg Gynecol Obstet 90:752–760, 1950.
3. Bricker EM: Bladder substitution after pelvic evisceration. Surg Clin North Am 30:1511–1521, 1950.
4. Kock NG, Nilson AE, Nilsson LO, et al: Urinary diversion via a continent ileal reservoir: Clinical results in 12 patients. J Urol 128:469–475, 1982.
5. Kock NG, Nilson AE, Norlen LJ, et al: Changes in renal parenchyma and the upper urinary tracts following urinary diversion via a continent ileum reservoir. An experimental study in dogs. Scand J Urol Nephrol 49(5):11, 1978.
6. Penalver MA, Bejany DE, Averette HE, et al: Continent urinary diversion in gynecologic oncology. Gynecol Oncol 34:274–288, 1989.
7. Rowland RG, Mitchell ME, Bihrle R, et al: Indiana continent urinary reservoir. J Urol 137:1136–1139, 1987.

13

Repair of Vesicovaginal Fistulas and Operative Injuries to the Distal Ureter

Most injuries to the lower urinary tract occur during the course of gynecologic-related procedures, usually hysterectomy. An unrecognized bladder injury will result in fistula formation. In the United States, reports in the last two decades indicate that over 80 per cent of injuries to the bladder are associated with gynecologic surgery. Vesicovaginal fistulas associated with hysterectomy are predominantly associated with abdominal procedures. For instance, in the recent Mayo Clinic report of 156 such fistulas (1988), 85 per cent were associated with abdominal hysterectomies, 13 per cent with vaginal hysterectomies, and only 2 per cent with radical hysterectomies.[7] Distal ureteral injuries are most often encountered during surgery for large adherent pelvic masses, intraligamentous leiomyomata, induration of pericervical tissue due to infection or cancer, endometriosis, and prior pelvic radiation therapy.

Over 95 per cent of vesicovaginal fistulas can be repaired using a vaginal approach. Absolute indications for an abdominal approach include complex fistulas involving the bowel, uterus, or ureters; inaccessible location of the fistula; or the presence of a contracted bladder that may require augmentation. Relative indications for abdominal closure include multiple prior repairs, fistulas associated with x-ray therapy, or excessive vaginal scarring.

A vaginal approach used for small to medium-sized fistulas is the Latzko procedure. Some large fistulas may require an abdominal approach, but many can be closed transvaginally. All fistulas require adequate mobilization, and adequate mobilization of the bladder is extremely important to ensure closure without tension. Most fistula surgeons do not excise the tract, and it is simply invaginated during repair. A ureteral catheter should be placed prior to surgical intervention if the ureteral orifices are within 1 cm of the fistula or if the fistula is sufficiently large that the integrity of the ureter might be compromised during repair. Systemic or topical estrogen should be given for at least 3 weeks prior to repair in postmenopausal women or women who are estrogen deficient for other reasons. All patients are placed on prophylactic antibiotics. In menstruating women, the time chosen for surgical intervention should be well away from the menstrual period, because of engorgement of tissues during menstruation.

For distal ureteral injuries within 4 to 6 cm of the ureterovesical junction, a ureteroneocystostomy is usually employed. One must adhere to the time-honored principles of repair. These include maintenance of hemostasis, using a limited number of sutures to avoid necrosis, ureteral catheterization, retroperitoneal drainage, and absolute lack of tension at the anastomotic site.

Pathophysiologic changes from either repair of vesicovaginal fistula or ureteroneocystostomy revolve around necrosis at the anastomosis site or hematoma formation with subsequent reformation of the fistula. Therefore, sutures should be kept to a minimum, and the bladder should be drained with transurethral or suprapubic catheterization. Additionally, in ureteral repair, the retroperitoneal space should be drained. Reflux can be a problem for patients undergoing ureteroneocystostomy.

Text continued on page 206

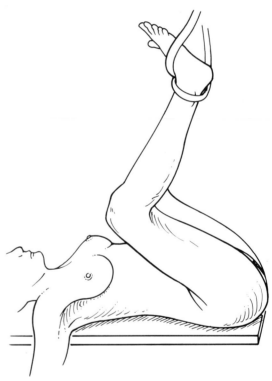

Figure 13–1. Positioning of the patient is critical for adequate exposure. For the Latzko procedure, the exaggerated lithotomy position with moderate Trendelenburg tilt gives adequate exposure in most patients. The exaggerated lithotomy position implies that the patient's buttocks protrude over the end of the table. About 15 degrees of Trendelenburg tilt will allow the anterior vaginal wall to appear perpendicular to the surgeon's line of vision. For large fistulas, better exposure may be achieved by placing the patient in the prone position with the ankles raised by stirrups (the Lawson position).

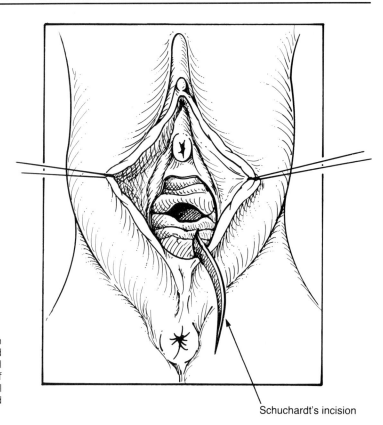

Schuchardt's incision

Figure 13-2. Schuchardt's incision. In patients with small caliber vaginas, a Schuchardt's incision should be employed. The incision is similar to a medial lateral episiotomy and is carried from an area near the site of the fistula downward and lateral to the anus. Bilateral Schuchardt's incisions may occasionally be needed for adequate exposure.

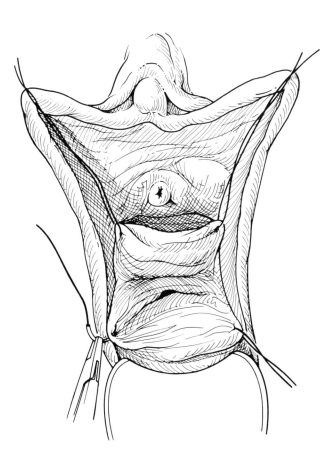

Figure 13-3. The Latzko partial colpocleisis. This type of repair may be used for small to medium-sized fistulas located high in the vagina, which are usually associated with hysterectomy. Occasionally, cephalad fistulas high in the vault following radiation therapy may be closed with this method. One disadvantage of this method is the slight foreshortening of the vagina that may occur. Large labia may be stitched laterally. Four-quadrant traction sutures of 0 polypropylene are placed in the healthy vaginal wall about 3 to 4 cm from the fistula edge. These traction sutures allow one to pull the fistula to the operating field. An alternate method is to place a small Foley catheter through the fistulous tract to allow one to pull the fistula to the field.

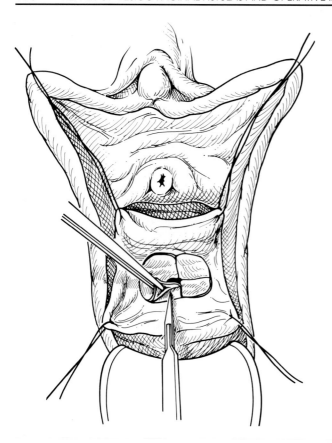

Figure 13–4. The area around the fistula is injected with vasopressin (Pitressin), 10 units (one ampule) in 50 ml saline, to facilitate dissection and decrease blood loss. A circular incision that includes only the vaginal mucosa is made. The 2- to 3-cm circular area is then divided into quadrants. Using a No. 11 blade, and beginning in the posterior quadrants, the vaginal mucosa is separated by sharp dissection from the underlying vaginal fascia. The fistula tract is not removed.

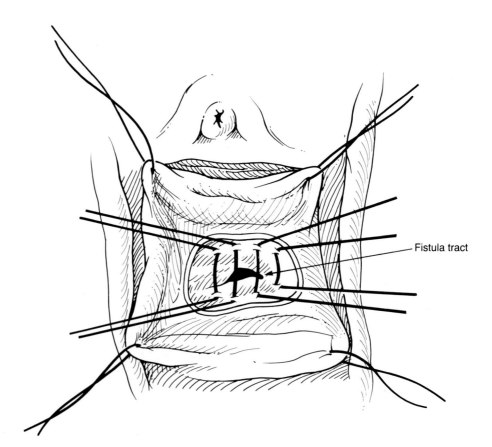

Fistula tract

Figure 13–5. The area over the fistula is closed in an inverted manner, using 3-0 polyglycolic acid suture. Three layers are used. All sutures are placed before they are tied, and sutures should be tied from lateral to medial.

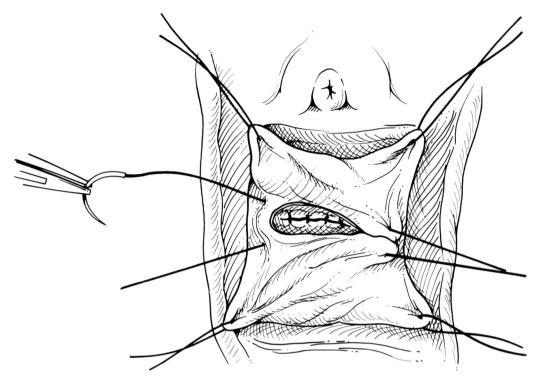

Figure 13-6. A second row of interrupted sutures with 3-0 polyglycolic acid has been placed. The third layer approximates the vaginal mucosa. The interrupted sutures are not tied until all sutures have been placed.

We prefer the use of a suprapubic catheter. The length of urinary drainage depends on the size of the fistula and the quality of tissues encountered during repair. These tissues heal slowly, and rarely is the period of drainage less than 10 days. Some surgeons require catheters only until the urine is grossly cleared of blood (as little as 2 to 3 days). A failed repair must be avoided, and a few extra days of catheterization can be tolerated by most patients. The patient is instructed to avoid coitus for 8 weeks.

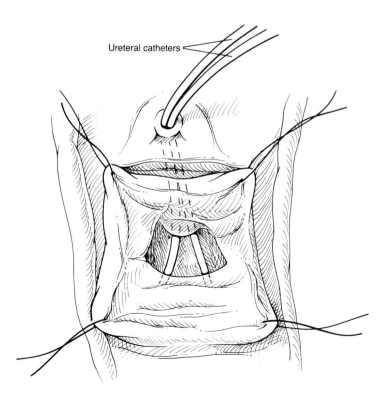

Ureteral catheters

Figure 13-7. A large fistula, as depicted here, usually requires ureteral catheterization to avoid injury during suturing of the vaginal mucosa. The ureteral catheters can be placed directly into the ureteral orifices and brought out through the urethra. Traction sutures may be used to improve exposure. After obtaining appropriate exposure, the junctional zone between the bladder and the vagina is incised.

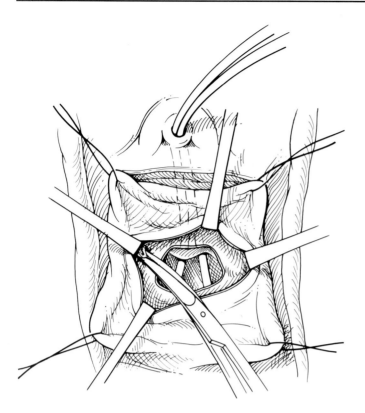

Figure 13–8. The key to a successful repair is adequate mobilization of tissues by use of a No. 11 blade or Mayo scissors. Special attention must be given to the lateral extensions of the fistulas. All palpable adhesive bands are carefully divided, regardless of the size of the fistula. Thus, flaps of vaginal tissue are created. Most fistula surgeons only freshen the tract; excision of the fistula is unnecessary. Countertraction is applied with Allis clamps as shown. In very large fistulas, to dissect the anterior and lateral fistula edges, entry into the space of Retzius from the vagina may be necessary. During the mobilization of the fistulous bed, one should not dissect too deeply toward the bladder in order to avoid perforation into the bladder.

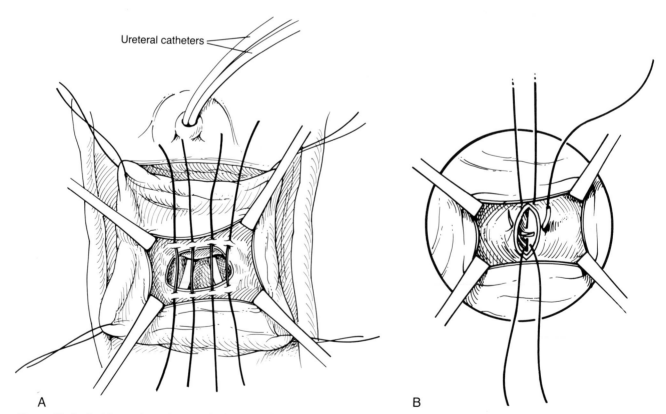

Ureteral catheters

A   B

Figure 13–9. *A*, After adequate mobilization, the bladder is closed in three layers. As noted, all sutures are initially placed beginning at the lateral edges. They are then tied. The fistula is not excised, but the rim of the fistula is inverted. Occasionally, it is easier to mobilize the bladder from lateral edge to lateral edge rather than anterior to posterior. In this instance, the bladder should be sutured vertically as noted in the inset (*B*). The bladder sutures should not be placed too close together to avoid tissue perfusion disturbance and necrosis.

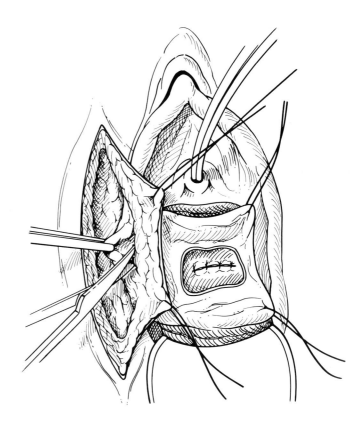

Figure 13–10. Martius bulbocavernosus flap. To bolster large fistulas, a bulbocavernosus or other local grafts from the gracilis muscle or portions of the gluteus maximus may be used. The simplest of these is the Martius, and adequate tissue is available in most patients. An incision is made over the bulbocavernosus bundle, and the tissue is mobilized. A Martius-type graft adds support to the urethra and bulk to the bladder neck and bladder base. Additionally, it decreases and/or obliterates the dead space between vaginal mucosa and bladder and may bring in a new blood supply to an area of poor vascularity.

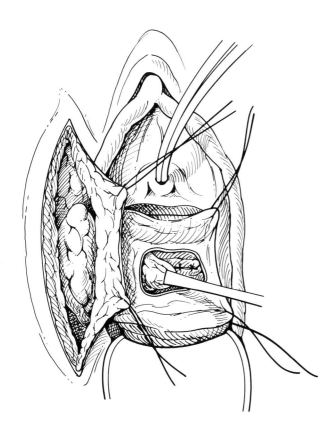

Figure 13–11. The labial fat pad and graft have been sectioned anteriorly and brought in to cover the previously placed two-layer closure of the bladder fistula. Because of its blood supply from the external pudendal and the internal pudendal arteries, the labial fat pad can be mobilized from anterior or posterior.

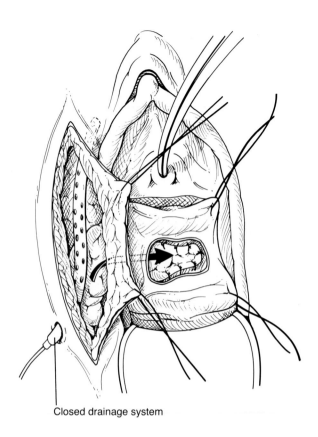

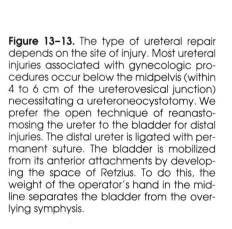

Closed drainage system

Figure 13–12. The labial fat pad graft is sutured over the second layer of bladder closure, using 3-0 polyglycolic interrupted sutures. A closed drainage system such as a Jackson-Pratt or Blake is placed subcutaneously in the previous incision over the fat pad area. The vaginal mucosa can be closed transversely or vertically over the inserted fat pad. With radiation-induced fistulas, one can use a modified bulbocavernosus myocutaneous flap, as suggested by Hoskins and colleagues.[5]

The suprapubic catheter should be left in place for a minimum of 2 weeks. We prefer to use a loosely placed vaginal pack for 48 hours, particularly when some type of graft is used. If ureteral catheters are utilized, they should be left in for 7 to 10 days.

Figure 13–13. The type of ureteral repair depends on the site of injury. Most ureteral injuries associated with gynecologic procedures occur below the midpelvis (within 4 to 6 cm of the ureterovesical junction) necessitating a ureteroneocystotomy. We prefer the open technique of reanastomosing the ureter to the bladder for distal injuries. The distal ureter is ligated with permanent suture. The bladder is mobilized from its anterior attachments by developing the space of Retzius. To do this, the weight of the operator's hand in the midline separates the bladder from the overlying symphysis.

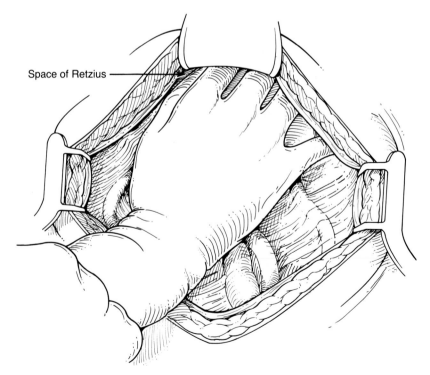

Space of Retzius

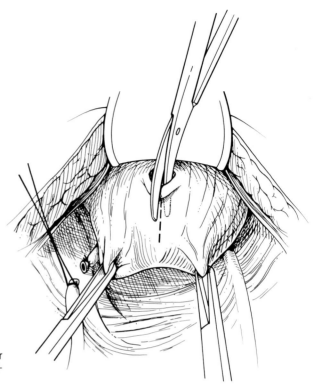

Figure 13–14. A vertical incision is made in the dome of the bladder beginning in the space of Retzius. The distal ureter has been ligated.

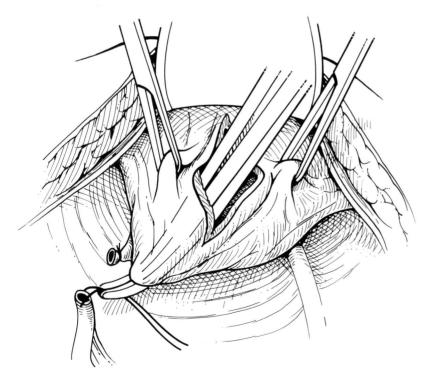

Figure 13–15. A small incision is made on the ipsilateral side of injury in the dome of the bladder, and a fine-tipped clamp is pushed through the serosa. The ureter is brought into the bladder.

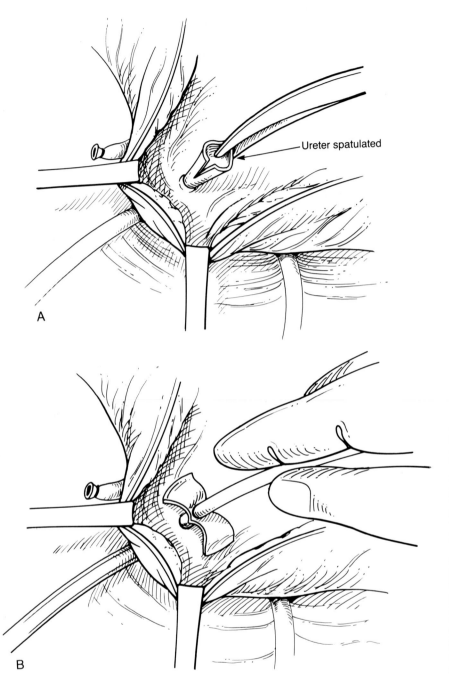

Ureter spatulated

A

B

Figure 13–16. *A,* Once the ureter is brought into the bladder, it is spatulated. A 6 to 8 French pediatric feeding tube or single J ureteral catheter is placed retrograde up the ureter to the renal pelvis *(B).* If a single J ureteral catheter is unavailable, we prefer to place a 4-0 chromic suture through the ureter and the pediatric feeding tube at the level of the pelvic brim to ensure the splint is not displaced by ureteral peristalsis.

The use of a submucosal tunnel is controversial and may not be needed for the adult urinary tract system. Some have noted more long-term complications in patients who had a tunneling procedure compared with those who had direct implantation. Tunneling is time consuming in an emergency situation. It requires a relatively long ureter, and its use may result in scarring.

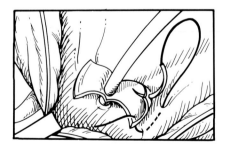

Figure 13–17. The spatulated ureteral ends are sutured to the bladder mucosa and muscularis with a 4-0 polyglycolic acid suture using a mattress technique.

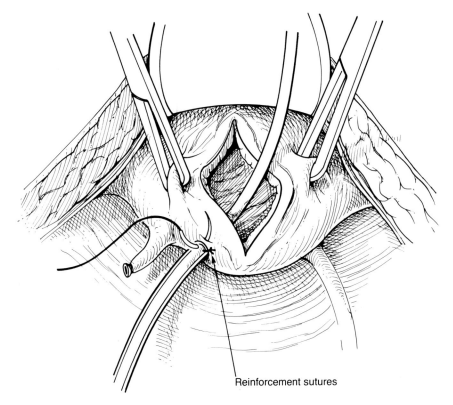

Figure 13–18. Three or four sutures of 3-0 nylon or polypropylene are placed through the outside bladder wall and the adventitia of the ureter at the anastomotic site to ensure stability and a tension-free anastomosis. The ureteral catheter is brought out through a separate stab wound in the bladder and abdominal wall and tied to a suprapubic catheter. The ureteral and suprapubic catheters are removed in 10 to 14 days in nonirradiated patients. A closed drainage system is placed at the site of the anastomosis and brought out through a separate stab wound.

Reinforcement sutures

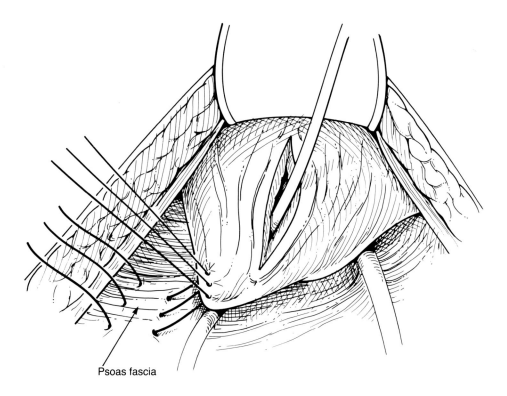

Psoas fascia

Figure 13–19. When the ureteral injury is below the pelvic brim and the ureter appears too short for tension-free anastomosis, the psoas muscle hitch for the mobilized bladder can be used. Three or four permanent sutures of 3-0 polypropylene are used to attach the seromuscular layer of the bladder to the ipsilateral psoas muscle belly fascia.

When a long segment of distal ureter is involved, the gap can be bridged by utilizing a flap from the bladder as described in the Boari-Ockerblad method. The Demel technique (bladder splitting) is an excellent alternative, is less prone to stricture development, and is our flap of choice.

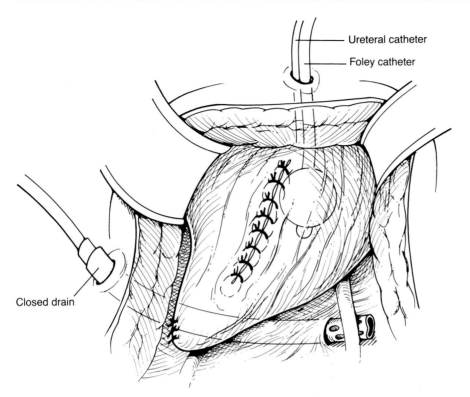

Figure 13–20. The bladder is closed in two layers with a running 3-0 chromic suture and followed by an interrupted 3-0 polyglycolic acid suture. The ureteral catheter is brought out through a separate stab wound along with the suprapubic catheter. A Jackson-Pratt or Blake drain is placed at the anastomotic site.

POTENTIAL PROBLEM AREAS

For large vesicovaginal fistulas, the ureter should be catheterized preoperatively in order to avoid injury. Hemostasis should be meticulously maintained, and tissues should be approximated with absolute lack of tension. Bladder catheterization is indicated for a period of 7 to 10 days postoperatively, depending on the size and cause of the fistula. Patients with radiation-induced fistulas or multiple prior repairs may require a longer period of catheterization. When the ureter is reapproximated to the dome of the bladder, hemostasis must be maintained, and a minimal number of sutures utilized. A tension-free anastomosis must be ensured by using serosa-to-serosa sutures of the ureter to the bladder. Additional steps to ensure a tension-free anastomosis might include psoas hitch, the use of a Boari flap, or the Demel bladder-splitting technique.

REFERENCES

1. Demel R: Plastic reconstruction of ureter from bladder. Zentralbl Chir 51:2008, 1924.

2. Elkins TE, Drescher C, Martey JO, Fort D: Vesicovaginal fistula revisited. Obstet Gynecol 72:307, 1988.

3. Elkins TE, DeLancey JOL, McGuire EJ: The use of modified Martius graft as an adjunctive technique in vesicovaginal and rectovaginal fistula repair. Obstet Gynecol 75:727, 1990.

4. Harrow BR: A neglected maneuver for uretero-vesical implantation following injury at gynecologic operations. J Urol 100:280, 1968.

5. Hoskins WJ, Park RC, Long R, et al: Repair of urinary tract fistulas with bulbocavernous flaps. Obstet Gynecol 63:580, 1984.

6. Latzko W: Postoperative vesicovaginal fistulas: Genesis and therapy. Am J Surg 58:211, 1942.

7. Lee RA, Symmonds RE, Williams TJ: Current status of genitourinary fistula. Obstet Gynecol 71:313, 1988.

8. McCall ML, Bolten KA (trans and ed): Martius' Gynecologic Operations: With Emphasis on Topographic Anatomy. Little, Brown, Boston, 1957, pp 322–333.

9. Moir C: Vesicovaginal fistula. Thoughts on treatment of 350 cases. Proc R Soc Med 59:1019, 1966.

10. Ockerblad NE: Reimplantation of the ureter into the bladder by a flap method. J Urol 57:845, 1947.

11. Symmonds RE: Ureteral injuries associated with gynecologic surgery: Prevention and management. Clin Obstet Gynecol 19:623, 1976.

14

Rectovaginal Fistula

The two general categories for etiology of rectovaginal fistula are congenital and acquired. By far, the majority of fistulas encountered by the gynecologic surgeon are of the acquired type. In this category, about half are due to obstetrical injuries and one fourth to operative gynecologic trauma (abdominal and vaginal hysterectomies, posterior repairs, etc.); the remainder are due to radiation injury, inflammatory bowel disease, and other types of trauma and infectious processes.

Work-up of these patients includes a detailed history and physical examination to establish the size and location of the fistula, whether single or multiple, the status of the sphincter, and the presence of underlying processes, for example, neoplasia, inflammatory condition, radiation injury, or infection. Upper gastrointestinal (GI) series with small bowel follow-through, barium enema, flexible sigmoidoscopy and colonoscopy, intravenous pyelography (IVP), and fistulography can be of invaluable help in the most complex cases.

There are several classifications of rectovaginal fistulas depending on location, size, and etiology. A practical classification is to consider three types, depending on location: (1) low, where the fistula is situated at or just above the dentate line; (2) high, where the fistula involves the posterior fornix and probably coincides with that portion of the vagina lined internally by peritoneum; and (3) middle, where its position lies between low (1) and high (2). An anovaginal fistula—when the opening in the rectum is below the dentate line—is included in this atlas as a subclassification of low rectovaginal fistulas because the approach to their treatment is similar.

There are no pathophysiologic changes.

POTENTIAL RISKS

During repair of low rectovaginal fistulas, the sphincter ani needs to be mobilized widely. Extreme care should be exercised not to injure the inferior hemorrhoidal nerve and vessels, which enter the muscle on its lateral and posterior third. It is recommended to preserve the scar tissue that joins together the edges of the severed sphincter, because this increases the "holding power" of the sutures during repair. Hematomas and infection are dreaded complications that should be kept to a minimum by good surgical technique.

OPERATIVE TECHNIQUES

Timing of repair of rectovaginal fistulas, and indeed of fistulas in general, is a matter of some controversy. Some advocate immediate repair, whereas others favor a waiting period (months) during which a number of fistulas will heal spontaneously, depending on etiology and aggressive medical management. Once the decision for operative intervention has been made, the bowel is prepared with one of the available protocols. We favor the insertion of a central line (triple lumen) to keep the bowel at rest for 10 to 14 days after surgery (medical colostomy).

POSTOPERATIVE CARE

The patient is started on hyperalimentation for about 7 to 10 days. Oral intake is not permitted except for water. Beginning on the seventh day, enteral feeding is initiated with half-strength protein hydrolysate, 1000 ml a day, and increased to full strength in 48 hours. The Foley catheter that was inserted after surgery is removed on the second day. Stool softeners are prescribed before the patient leaves the hospital. Full oral feeding is allowed by the 14th day after surgery. Sexual activity is delayed for 4 to 6 weeks.

LOW RECTOVAGINAL FISTULA

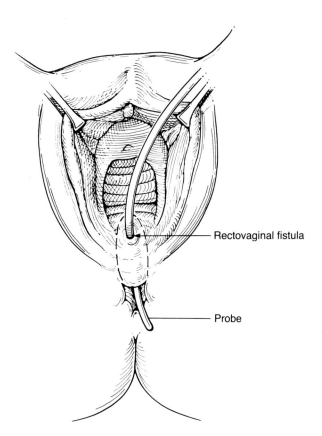

— Rectovaginal fistula

— Probe

Figure 14–1. The majority, if not all, of these fistulas are repaired by converting them to a ''complete perineal tear'' (fourth degree obstetrical laceration). With a probe in the fistula, an incision is made from anus to vagina to encompass the whole length of the fistulous tract.

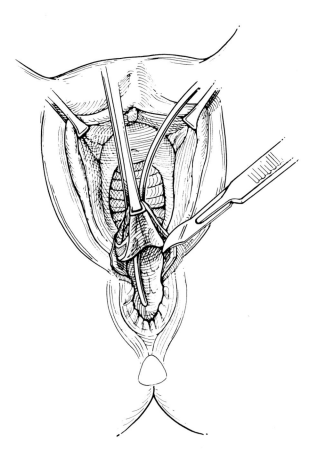

Figure 14–2. The fistulous tract and the scar tissue surrounding it are removed by sharp dissection.

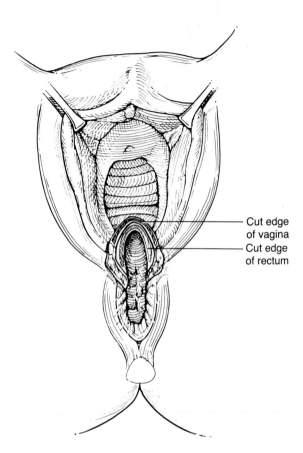

Figure 14–3. After removing the fistula, the surgeon should recognize the different structures that form the perineal body and rectovaginal septum.

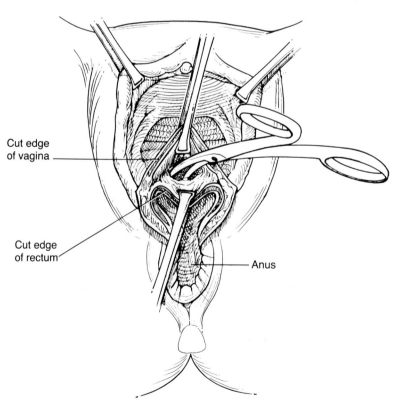

Figure 14–4. The vagina is separated from the rectum high enough into the avascular rectovaginal space to allow the surgeon to close the rectum without tension.

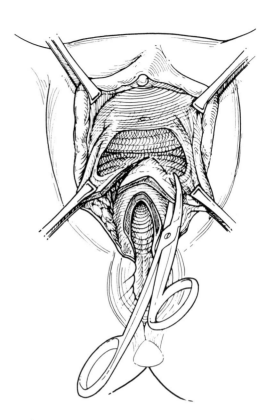

Figure 14–5. The scar tissue of the distal vagina is removed at this time, facilitating, by improving exposure, the next steps of the operation.

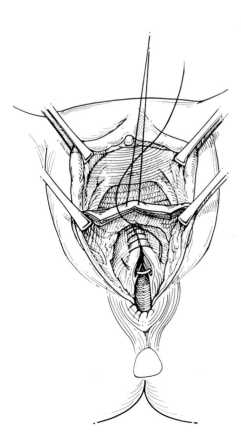

Figure 14–6. Repair of the rectal mucosa and internal sphincter is performed in one layer with running or interrupted 4–0 polyglycolic suture. Alternatively, it may be done in two layers.

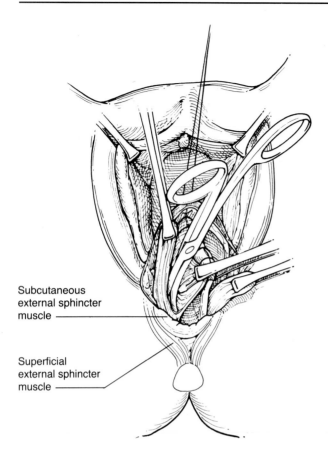

Subcutaneous
external sphincter
muscle

Superficial
external sphincter
muscle

Figure 14–7. The external sphincter is dissected, with care taken not to disturb the inferior hemorrhoidal nerve, which enters the muscle on its posterior third. It is also important to preserve part of the scar tissue on each end of the transected sphincter to facilitate its approximation during sphincteroplasty.

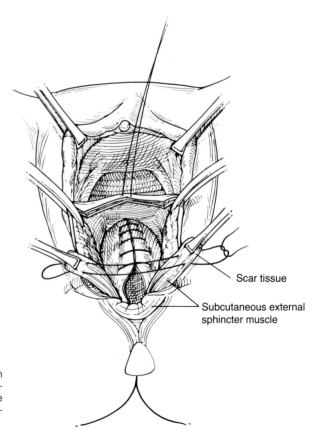

Scar tissue

Subcutaneous external
sphincter muscle

Figure 14–8. The sphincter is repaired by imbricating the muscle with four interrupted stitches of 2–0 polyglycolic acid sutures using the far-near, near-far technique. The free end is sutured to the belly of the imbricated muscle with one or two through-and-through polyglycolic acid stitches.

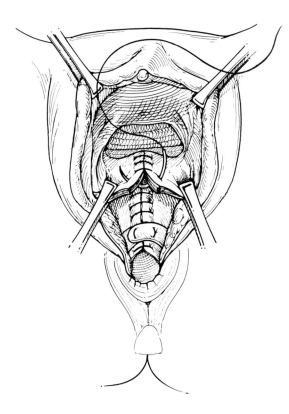

Figure 14–9. The remainder of the rectum has been closed. The vaginal edges are approximated to the level of the hymenal ring with a continuous or interrupted suture of 2–0 polyglycolic material.

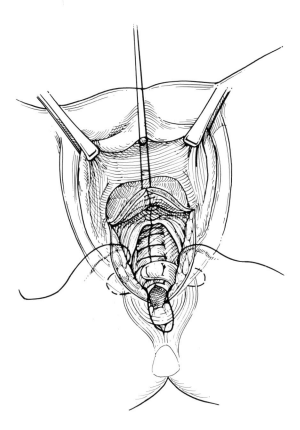

Figure 14–10. A ``reinforcement stitch'' is placed just above and lateral to the sphincter in a position normally occupied by the superficial transverse perineal muscle.

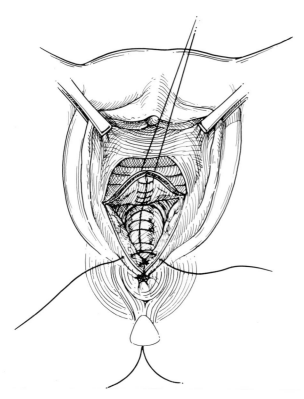

Figure 14–11. Once the ''reinforcement stitch'' is tied, the procedure is essentially converted to a perineoplasty. The skin is approximated over the sphincter by a ''single'' interrupted or running suture of absorbable polyglycolic acid material.

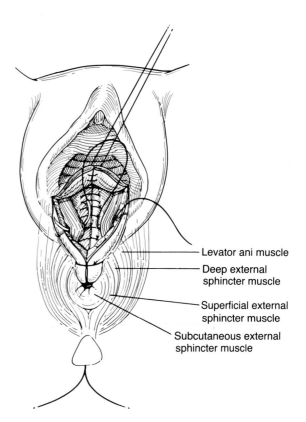

Levator ani muscle

Deep external
sphincter muscle

Superficial external
sphincter muscle

Subcutaneous external
sphincter muscle

Figure 14–12. The deeper layer of the perineal body, the levator ani, is brought together in the midline by interrupted ''figures of eight'' sutures of 2–0 polyglycolic acid material.

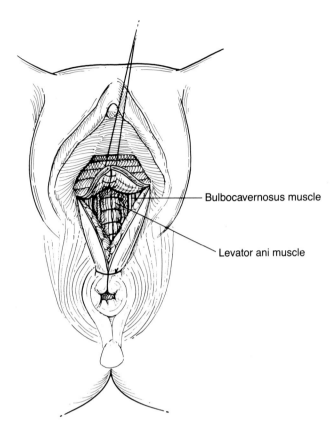

Bulbocavernosus muscle

Levator ani muscle

Figure 14–13. The deeper layer of the perineal body has been completed.

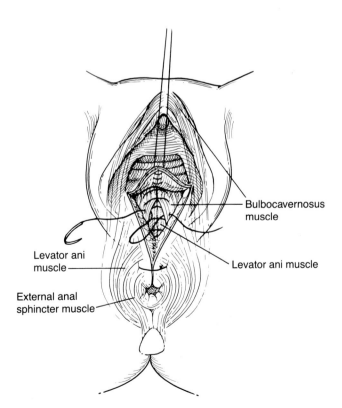

Bulbocavernosus muscle

Levator ani muscle

Levator ani muscle

External anal sphincter muscle

Figure 14–14. The beginning of the approximation of the superficial layer of the perineal body, the bulbocavernosus.

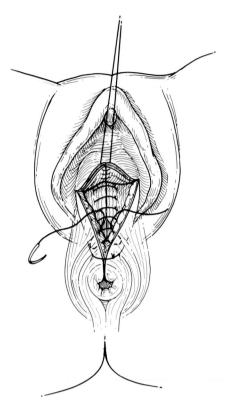

Figure 14–15. The superficial layer of the perineal body has been completed.

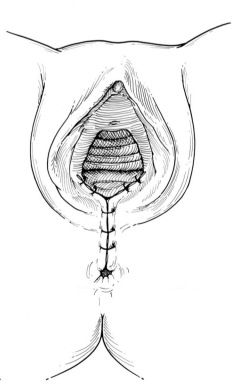

Figure 14–16. Closure of the vestibule and perineal skin.

MID RECTOVAGINAL FISTULA

Fistulas in the mid-portion of the vagina, if uncomplicated by an underlying process (radiation, ulcerative disorders), can be closed via rectum or vagina with a high degree of success. The vaginal approach is demonstrated here.

MID RECTOVAGINAL FISTULA

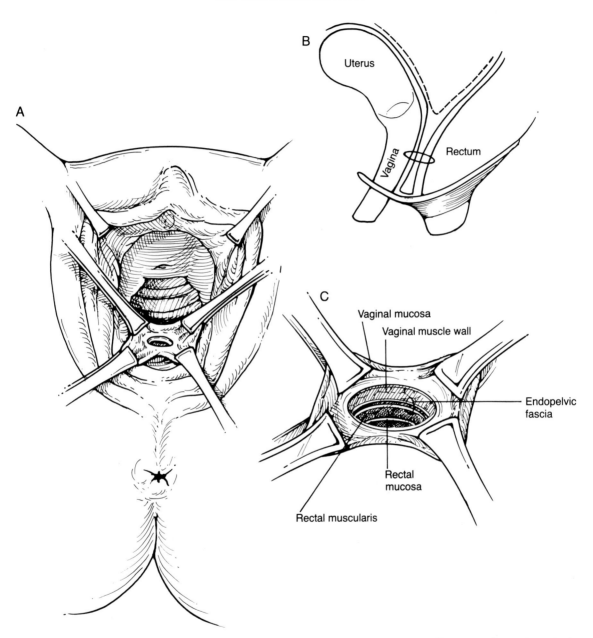

Figure 14–17. *A,* A circular incision is made around the fistula 5 mm or more from its edges. The avascular rectovaginal space is entered, and the vagina is separated from the rectum for at least 2 cm so that further steps in the operation can be performed without undue tension. *B,* The location of the endopelvic fascia proper relative to both vagina and rectum. *C,* The fistulous tract has been resected and the different layers from vagina to rectum are diagrammatically shown.

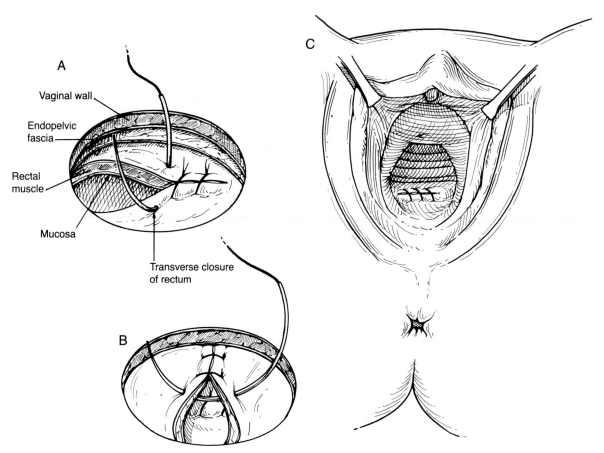

Figure 14–18. *A,* The rectal mucosa is approximated transversely with 3–0 polyglycolic sutures. The endopelvic fascia and the muscularis are closed next with similar sutures. Alternatively, the rectum can be closed in one layer. *B,* The endopelvic fascia and the muscularis of the vagina are closed in a vertical fashion with 3–0 polyglycolic sutures. *C,* The vaginal mucosa is closed transversely to prevent narrowing and to promote better function.

HIGH RECTOVAGINAL FISTULA

Almost without exception, approach to these fistulas is through the abdominal route. The majority of fistulas encountered by the gynecologist are due to operative injury encountered during repair of a high rectocele, enterocele, and culdoplasty. Radiation fistulas are more complex in management, and the procedures utilized for their correction are beyond the scope of this atlas.

Following adequate bowel preparation, the abdomen is entered through a transverse muscle-splitting or vertical incision. The abdomen is routinely explored before the surgeon directs attention to the pelvis.

HIGH RECTOVAGINAL FISTULA

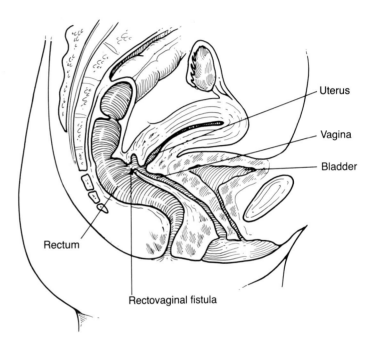

Figure 14–19. The most common location of high rectovaginal fistula and its relation to neighboring structures.

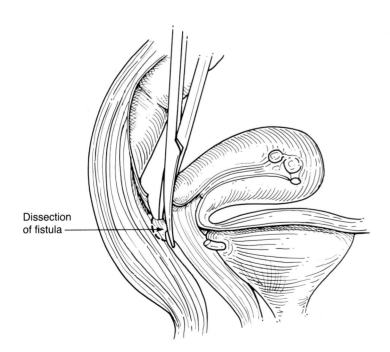

Figure 14–20. The rectum is separated from the vagina for a distance of several centimeters into the avascular rectovaginal space.

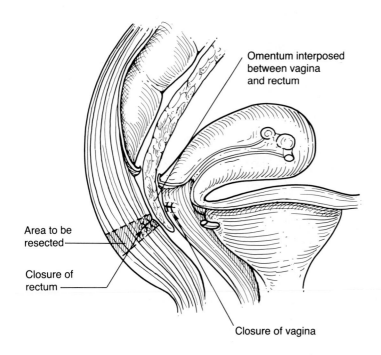

Omentum interposed
between vagina
and rectum

Area to be
resected

Closure of
rectum

Closure of vagina

Figure 14-21. Depending on the local condition of the tissues, the fistula in the rectosigmoid can be excised and the defect closed in two layers with 2–0 polyglycolic acid sutures. The vagina is likewise closed, interposing omentum to enhance healing and prevent apposition of suture lines.

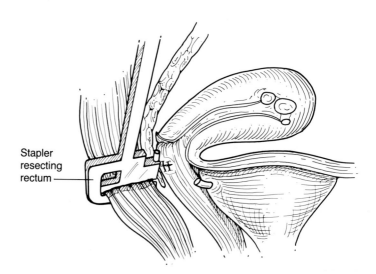

Stapler
resecting
rectum

Figure 14-22. The rectosigmoid is often involved in a chronic inflammatory process and requires resection to ensure better healing and success. The GIA (gastrointestinal anastomosis) stapler or the thoracoabdominal stapler can be used for the resection.

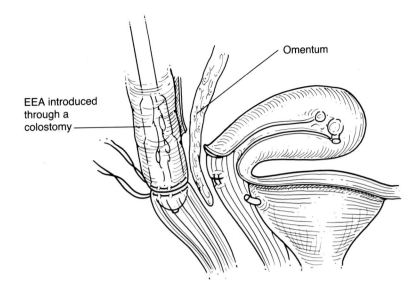

Figure 14–23. The rectosigmoid can be reanastomosed in two layers with suture material or with staples as illustrated here using the EEA (end-to-end anastomosis) stapler. The anastomosis has been completed. Omentum has been anchored between the vagina and rectum to reinforce the anastomosis and ensure better healing.

REFERENCES

Corman M: Anal incontinence following obstetrical injury. Dis Colon Rectum 28(2):86–89, 1983.

Corman ML: Anal Incontinence in Colon and Rectal Surgery, 2nd ed., JB Lippincott, Philadelphia, 1989, chap 5, pp 171–207.

Given FT: Rectovaginal fistula. Am J Obstet Gynecol 108(1):41–45, 1970.

Goldberg SM, Gordon PH, Nivatvongs S: Essentials of Ano-Rectal Surgery. JB Lippincott, Philadelphia, 1980, pp 286–287.

Gordon PH: Rectovaginal fistula. In Gordon PH, Nivatvongs S (eds): Principles and Practices of Surgery for the Colon, Rectum and Anus. St. Louis, MI, Quality Medical Publishing, 1992, chap 16, pp 361–381.

Hagihara PF, Griffen WO Jr: Delayed correction of ano-rectal incontinence due to anal sphincteral injury. Arch Surg 111:63–66, 1976.

Rosenshein NB, Genadry RR, Woodruff JD, et al: An anatomic classification of rectovaginal septal defects. Am J Obstet Gynecol 137(4):439–442, 1980.

15

The Use of Locally Mobilized Skin (Z-Plasty and Rhomboid Flaps) for Large Defects

Deborah L. Coleman Gallup, M.D.

Carcinoma of the vulva often involves the labia or clitoris. Approximately 13 per cent arise on the perineum or posterior fourchette, although 41 per cent may involve this region. Numerous skin folds around the anterior vulva may allow for excision of the lesion, with the necessary 1.5- to 2-cm normal margin and relatively easy primary closure of an elliptical defect. However, large anterior, posterior, or posterolateral primary defects, when closed, are usually accompanied by tension at suture lines, resulting in wound breakdown. Frequently, they will require closure with local flaps. Surgical techniques using rhomboid skin flaps and Z-plasty are ideal for covering many of these defects.

Physiologic changes are minimal. The risk of urinary complications, bowel complications, or sexual dysfunction is minimized by adhering to principles of good surgical technique and aggressive postoperative care to prevent wound breakdown. Meticulous hemostasis is needed to prevent hematoma formation. To reduce the incidence of wound breakdown, suture lines must be tension free.

POTENTIAL PROBLEM AREAS

In addition to ensuring tension-free suture lines, a pressure dressing should be applied at the end of the procedure. An ice pack is used for at least 8 hours post procedure to lessen edema, which can also cause unwanted tension. If an extensive dissection is performed, loose vaginal packs should be inserted. The dressing and packs may be removed within 24 hours.

Patients should remain in bed for 3 to 5 days after procedures using large perineal flaps to allow partial healing. Thromboembolic prophylaxis utilizing the intermittent pressure cuffs or mini-dose heparin is essential. We prefer to use prophylactic, broad-spectrum antibiotics in these patients. Also, a Foley catheter is left in place for 24 hours to avoid urine spilling and pain at the suture lines. For anterior flaps, close to the urethra, the catheter may be left in place longer. Perineal toilet, with dilute povidone-iodine, should be given after each bowel movement. We prefer to apply collodion to suture lines as soon as bandages are removed. Sitz baths should be instituted as soon as the patient is ambulatory. Until that time, incision lines should be cleansed with a dilute hydrogen peroxide solution three times a day, followed by heat lamp treatment to ensure drying and then topical antibiotic ointment application. With posterior flaps, defecation should be delayed for 2 to 3 days until the flap has sealed to minimize infection. This is achieved by a low-residue diet and administration of Lomotil tablets. Stool softeners are used thereafter.

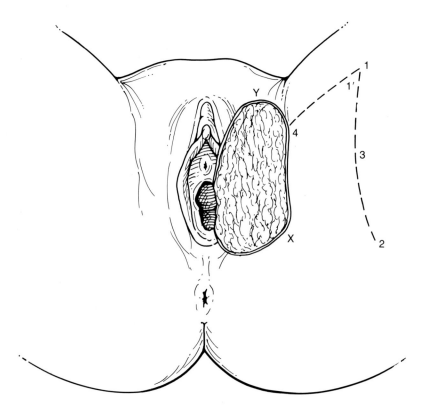

Figure 15–1. A large defect is shown. If after the vulvar lesion is excised the defect is too large to be closed primarily, a Z-plasty flap may be utilized. The length of the medial aspect of the defect should be measured. This length must be equal to the length of the proposed flap (line 1–2). The width of the flap (2 to the lateral edge of the defect) must also be wider than the length of the flap. Lengths shorter than this may interfere with the flap's blood supply, resulting in possible necrosis of the tip of the flap. Using meticulous hemostasis, flap incisions (1–2 and 1–4) should be extended through the skin and subcutaneous fat.

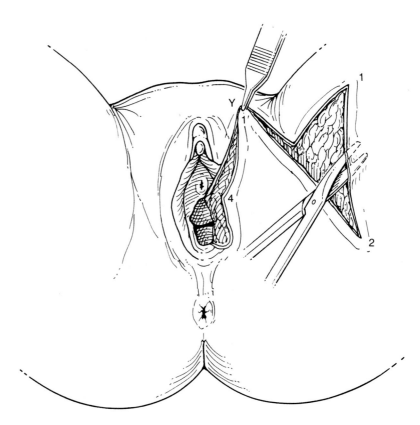

Figure 15–2. All adjacent tissue should be mobilized to release any undue tension. Metzenbaum scissors may be used to undermine the tissue adjacent to the flap as shown on the lateral portion. The apex of the flap, point 1', has been pulled to the apex of the defect, point Y.

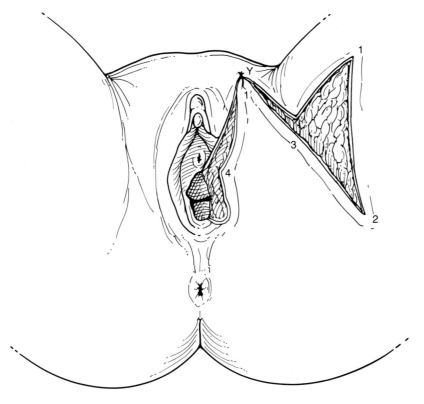

Figure 15–3. Using 3-0 or 4-0 monofilament polypropylene or nylon, point 1' should be sutured to the ventral aspect of the defect (apex). This stitch enters the skin of the ventral margin of the defect and then is brought through the flap with a subcuticular technique (see Fig. 15–4). The second suture should be placed in the posterior fourchette and be brought to the angle of the flap marked 4, with the same subcuticular technique. Then, point 3 should be sutured to the angle created by the entire Z-plasty.

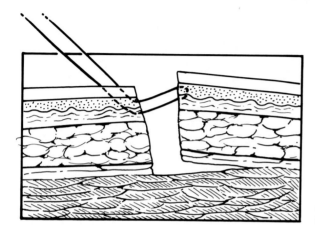

Figure 15–4. Modified mattress suture. Sutures are placed within the dermis and penetrate the skin on only one side of the incision. Knots should never be placed on the flap side.

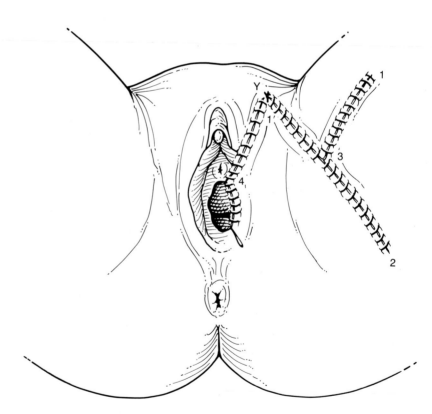

Figure 15–5. Remaining approximation of the flap to the adjacent skin can be performed in a number of ways. Stainless steel, inert skin clips cause very little tissue reaction, are preferred by some, and can be left in place for a long period of time. Nonabsorbable suture may give a slightly better cosmetic result. The subcuticular flap stitch can be employed throughout the entire closure. A pressure dressing is applied with fluffs, large pads, and elastic tape. These sutures will have to be removed when the wound edges have healed.

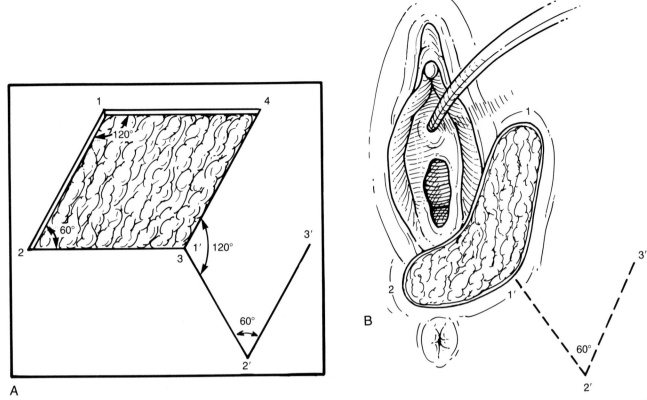

Figure 15–6. *A,* A skin defect in the shape of a rhomboid (1, 2, 3, 4) and a flap (1', 2', 3') are demonstrated. The angles formed by lines 1, 2, 3 and 1, 4, 3 are 60 degrees, and the angles formed by lines 2, 3, 4 and 2, 1, 4 are 120 degrees. One-centimeter deep incisions, 1', 2' and 2', 3', are made to create a skin flap to cover the defect. The length of 1, 2 is identical to 1', 2' and the length of 2, 3 is identical to 2', 3'. The angles in the flap also have to be the same as the defect. Angle 4, 1', 2 has to be the same as 4, 1, 2 and angle 1', 2', 3' has to be the same as 1, 2, 3. *B,* A large defect that crosses the midline. The line from 1' to 2' should be equal to the vertical length of the defect to be closed. The line from 3' to 2' should equal the horizontal length.

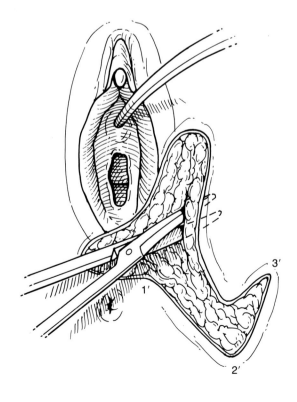

Figure 15–7. The flap is then undermined to mobilize the flap and release unwanted tension.

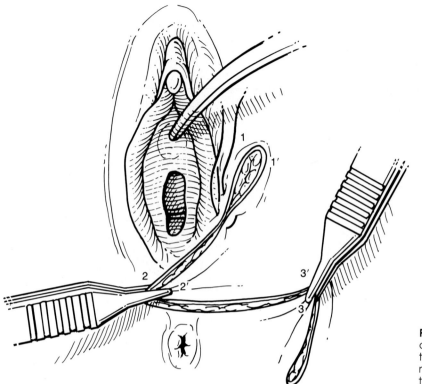

Figure 15–8. The flap is mobilized to cover the defect. Absorbable sutures can be used for the vaginal margins. We prefer 3-0 permanent monofilament suture for the flap area that covers the perineum.

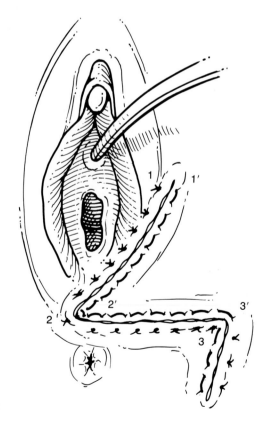

Figure 15–9. The defect is shown closed with interrupted sutures.

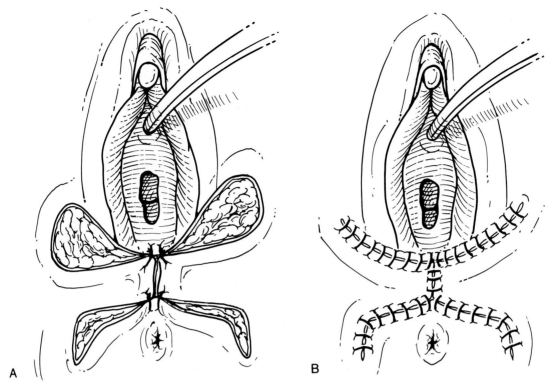

Figure 15–10. Bilateral rhomboid flaps have been created, mobilized, and sutured in the midline to cover a large perineal defect. *A* shows mobilization of the flaps to the midline after bilateral V incisions. *B,* The flaps are then sutured in place.

REFERENCES

1. Barnhill DR, Hoskins WJ, Metz P: Use of the rhomboid flap after partial vulvectomy. Obstet Gynecol 62:444, 1983.
2. Borges AF, Alexander SE: Relaxed skin tension lines, "Z" plasties on scars, and fusiform excision of lesion. Br J Plast Surg 15:242, 1962.
3. Jervis W, Salyer KE, Busquets MAV, Atkins RW: Further applications of the Limberg and Dufourmental flaps. Plast Reconstruct Surg 54:335, 1974.
4. Lister GD, Gibson T: Closure of rhomboid skin defects: The flaps of Limberg and Dufourmental. Br J Plast Surg 25:300, 1972.
5. McGregor IA: The theoretical basis of the Z-plasty. Br J Plast Surg 9:256, 1957.
6. Oneal RM, Dingman RO, Grabb WC: The teaching of plastic surgical techniques to medical students. Plast Reconstruct Surg 40:494, 1967.

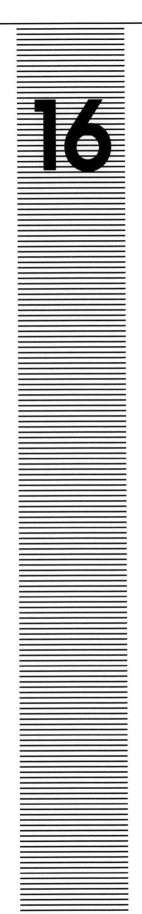

16

Gracilis Myocutaneous Flap

Reconstruction of the vagina following extensive pelvic surgery has been a surgical challenge for the physician and a major handicap for the patient. Faced with the loss of sexual function, a significant number of patients who otherwise would benefit by the procedure decline the operation. The introduction of myocutaneous flaps in plastic reconstructive procedures represents a major advance in surgery and provides the oncologic surgeon with a special "tool" to deal with the anatomic defects associated with ultra-radical surgery.

The gracilis myocutaneous flap is an expendable unit that is well suited for vaginal reconstruction. Thus there are no pathophysiologic changes. The resulting scars on the inner aspects of the thighs have not been a deterrent to the surgical procedure. Indeed, this procedure benefits not only the patient, by preserving sexual function, but also the surgeon, whom it provides with one of the better methods to reconstruct the pelvic floor following exenterative surgery.

POTENTIAL PROBLEM AREAS

The viability of the flap is dependent upon the preservation of the blood supply and on accurate delineation of its cutaneous territory. Points on technique are as follows: (1) proper identification of the muscle at its insertion, proximally or distally, will aid in the delineation of its cutaneous territory; (2) suture of the muscle to the subcuticular dermis will prevent disruption of the perforator vessels; (3) careful handling of the flaps will prevent spasm of the vascular pedicle with probable loss of skin; and (4) the distal third of the cutaneous territory is unreliable and should not be used unless "delaying techniques" are utilized.

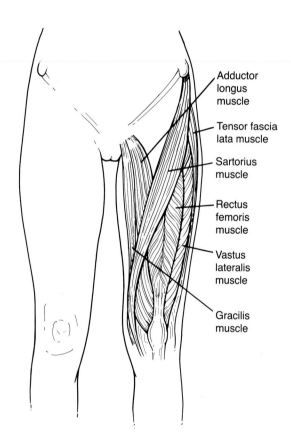

Adductor
longus
muscle

Tensor fascia
lata muscle

Sartorius
muscle

Rectus
femoris
muscle

Vastus
lateralis
muscle

Gracilis
muscle

Figure 16–1. Gracilis is one of a group of muscles (sartorius, rectus femoris, vastus lateralis, tensor fascia lata) that constitute the anterior compartment of the thigh. From its insertion in the symphysis pubis, it runs posterior to the adductor longus and sartorius muscle and anterior to the semimembranosus and semitendinosus to its insertion on the medial condyle of the knee.

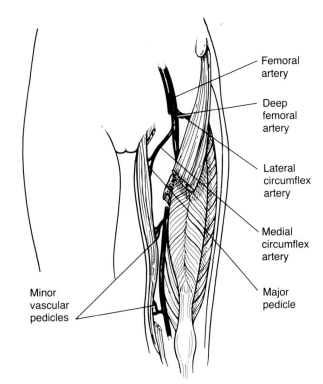

Figure 16–2. The vascular pedicle, branch of the medial circumflex artery, enters the muscle between 8 and 10 cm from the pubic tubercle. It represents the major blood supply and provides for an 8 × 20 cm flap elevation. On its distal third, the muscle has one or two pedicles that originate from the superficial femoral artery. They are sacrificed during flap elevation to provide for a good arc of rotation; however, the cutaneous territory on its distal third is unreliable and probably should not be used routinely. The sensory as well as the motor innervation of the flap is provided by a branch of the obturator nerve that enters the muscle at the same level as its vascular supply.

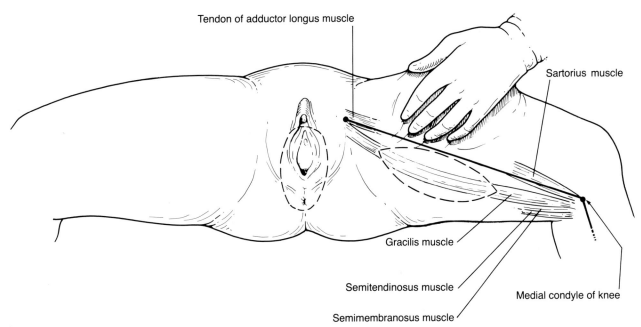

Figure 16–3. The cutaneous territory supported by the muscle must be defined accurately. The insertion of the adductor longus is easily identified at its origin because it is quite prominent with the leg abducted and rotated externally. The round tendon of the gracilis can be felt on the medial condyle of the knee. With a marking pen, these two points are jointed while putting upward traction on the skin. This maneuver affords correction for the tendency of the skin to sag downward.

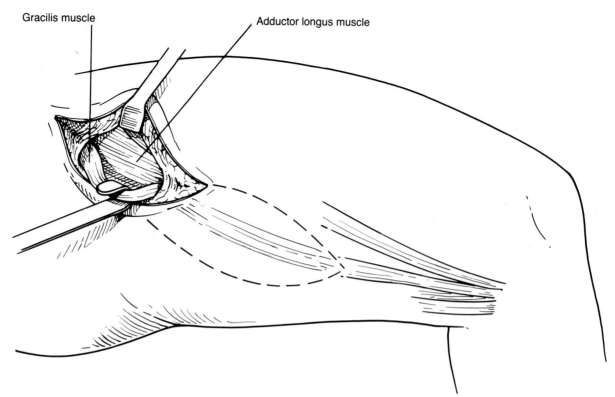

Figure 16–4. Proximal approach to identify the gracilis muscle. The incision is made on the anterior border of the flap and carried down to the fascia of the adductor longus. The saphenous vein is identified and kept anterior to the dissection. The fascia of the adductor longus is incised and the dissection is carried directly posteriorly. The gracilis is encountered and isolated. By keeping traction on the muscle, the cutaneous territory is outlined.

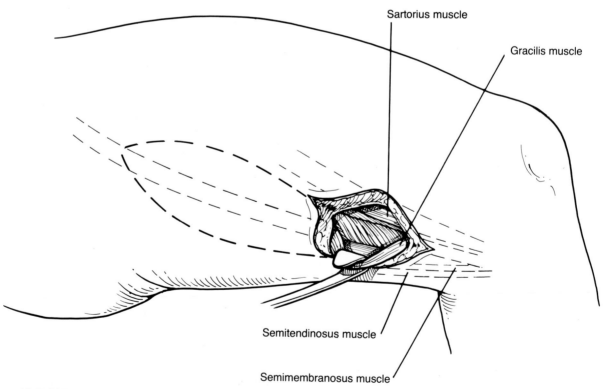

Figure 16–5. Distal approach to identify the gracilis muscle. An incision is made on the anterior border of the flap. The gracilis is recognized by the direction of the muscle fibers, which are horizontal and musculotendinous in nature. The sartorius, anteriorly, is muscular and the direction of its fibers is oblique at this level. A retractor is placed underneath the muscle and by applying traction, the cutaneous territory is outlined. Careful identification of the belly of the muscle is mandatory because the gracilis will support only the skin overlying the muscle 2 to 3 cm beyond its edge.

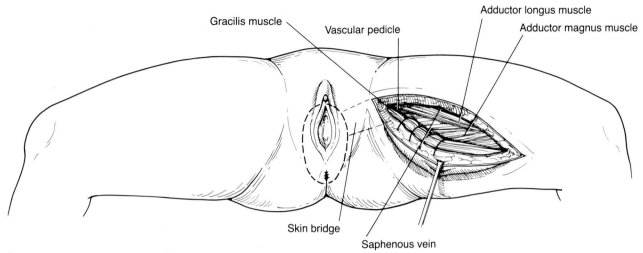

Figure 16–6. Once the surgeon is confident that the gracilis has been identified, the anterior border of the flap, throughout its length, is cut down to the fascia, exposing the adductor longus. The saphenous vein is recognized and kept anterior to the dissection. A few of its branches, as well as the minor vascular pedicles of the gracilis, are ligated. The muscle is sutured to the subcuticular dermis to prevent disruption of the perforator vessels and subsequent necrosis of the skin.

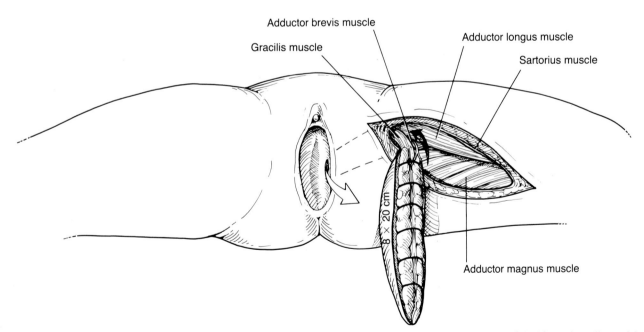

Figure 16–7. The main vascular pedicle is identified between the adductor longus and adductor brevis 8 to 10 cm from the pubic tubercle. They are carefully handled to prevent spasm. The posterior dissection can be completed quickly because there are no major structures that can be damaged in that area.

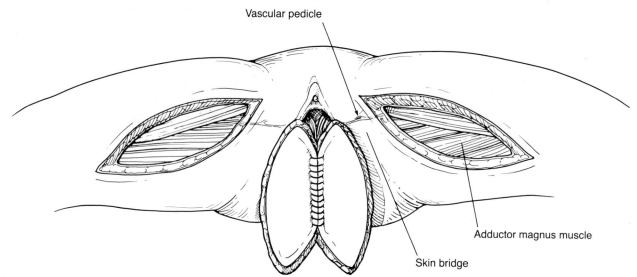

Figure 16–8. The proximal insertion of the muscle is not sectioned, but its fascia is, to facilitate rotation of the myocutaneous unit. For vaginal reconstruction following pelvic exenteration, the skin bridge between the thigh and the introitus is undermined wide enough to allow passage of the flaps with ease.

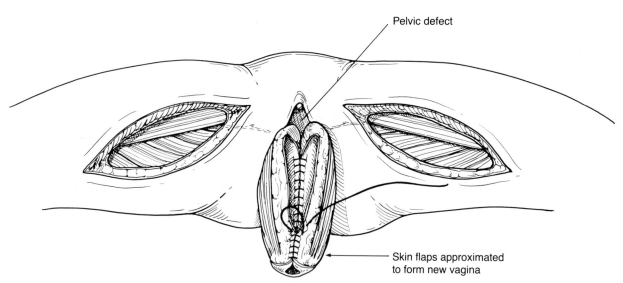

Figure 16–9. The flaps are approximated in the midline to create a neovaginal pouch.

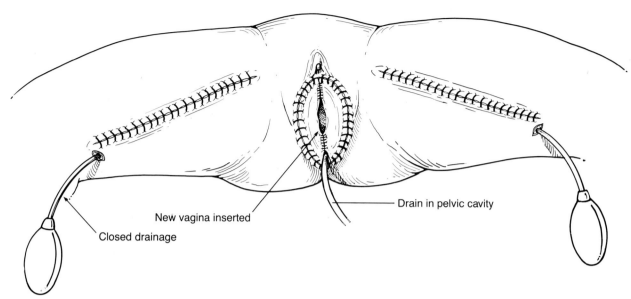

New vagina inserted

Closed drainage

Drain in pelvic cavity

Figure 16–10. The pouch is inserted into the pelvic defect and sutured to the perineal skin. The neovagina does not have to be fixed internally to prevent collapse. The defects on the thighs are sutured together. Closed drainage is employed for several days.

Bibliography

Becker DW Jr, Massey FM, McGraw JB: Musculo-cutaneous flaps in reconstructive pelvic surgery. Obstet Gynecol 54:178–183, 1979.

Franklin EW III, Bostwick J III, Burrell MO, Powell JL: Reconstructive techniques in radical pelvic surgery. Am J Obstet Gynecol 129:285–292, 1977.

Lacey CG, Stern JL, Feizenbaum S, et al: Vaginal reconstruction with use of gracilis myocutaneous flaps: The University of California, San Francisco, experience. Am J Obstet Gynecol 158:1278–1284, 1988.

McGraw JB, Massey FM, Shanklin KD, Horton CE: Vaginal reconstruction with gracilis myocutaneous flaps. Plast Reconstr Surg 58:176–183, 1976.

Morrow CP, Lacey CG, Lucas WE: Reconstructive surgery in gynecologic cancer employing the gracilis myocutaneous pedicle graft. Gynecol Oncol 7:176–187, 1979.

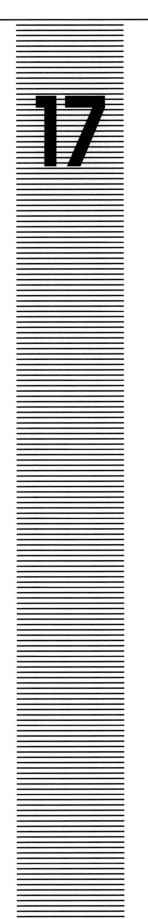

17

The Tensor Fascia Lata Flap

Laurel A. King, M.D.

En-bloc surgical resection of the vulva and inguinal nodes has been the mainstay of treatment for invasive vulvar carcinoma. The initial procedure, first described by Bassett in 1912[1] and later modified by Taussig[7] and Way,[9] was associated with a very high incidence of wound infection and dehiscence. In 1981, Hacker et al[4] described a modification of the groin incisions that significantly decreased the incidence of wound breakdown and wound infection. However, prolonged hospitalization resulting from wound infection and wound breakdown still occurs and is a very morbid and costly complication.

The catastrophic wound problems are thought to be secondary to the devascularization of tissue and large skin defects that occur with extensive resection, inherent to the operative procedure. The tensor fascia lata (TFL) flap, originally described in 1934, has been reported by several authors as a useful technique in covering large defects in the lower abdomen and inguinal, vulvar, perineal, and sacral areas.[2, 3, 5, 6, 8] Chafe and colleagues[2] reported decreased morbidity and a shorter postoperative course in patients who underwent an en bloc groin dissection and radical vulvectomy followed by bilateral TFL flaps.

The flap can be made as large as 25 cm in width × 40 cm in length. The TFL flap may be directly rotated into the defect or may be tunneled to the operative site. The distal border may extend within 5 to 8 cm of the knee.

PREOPERATIVE PATIENT PREPARATION

The patient should receive preoperative antibiotic prophylaxis. She should be informed that there will be numbness at the flap site. The patient may note some difficulty with ambulation, and physical therapy should be started when appropriate for her physical status and wound healing.

POTENTIAL PROBLEM AREAS

Care should be taken when elevating the flap to avoid disruption of the vascular pedicle. Care also must be taken not to strip the fascia lata away from its nutrient bed of subcutaneous tissue and skin. The fascia can be loosely approximated to the skin and subcutaneous tissue during flap elevation to prevent disruption of the fascia and loss of the blood supply to the flap. Care should be taken not to "bevel" the subcutaneous tissue during resection and narrow the undersurface of the flap. Care should also be taken at approximately 6 to 10 cm from the anterior iliac spine, where the flap is elevated, in order to avoid vascular pedicle disruption. If the patient is athletic and has prominent thigh musculature, the flap should be made approximately 5 cm longer than measured in order to compensate for the muscular bulk when the flap is rotated. Excessive muscle bulk will cause shortening of the flap when it is rotated.

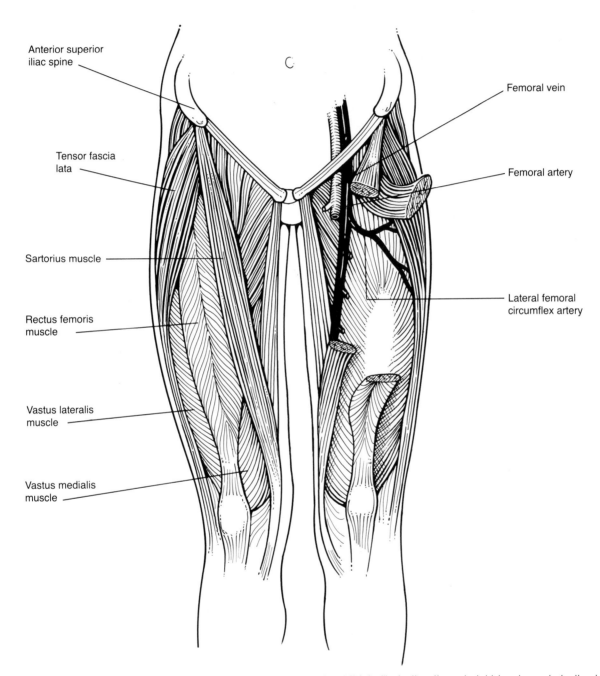

Anterior superior
iliac spine

Tensor fascia
lata

Sartorius muscle

Rectus femoris
muscle

Vastus lateralis
muscle

Vastus medialis
muscle

Femoral vein

Femoral artery

Lateral femoral
circumflex artery

Figure 17–1. Overview of muscular anatomy of the anterior and lateral thigh, illustrating the arterial blood supply to the tensor fascia lata (TFL) flap. The flap is supplied by branches of the lateral femoral circumflex artery. The vascular pedicle is located between the rectus femoris and vastus lateralis muscles.

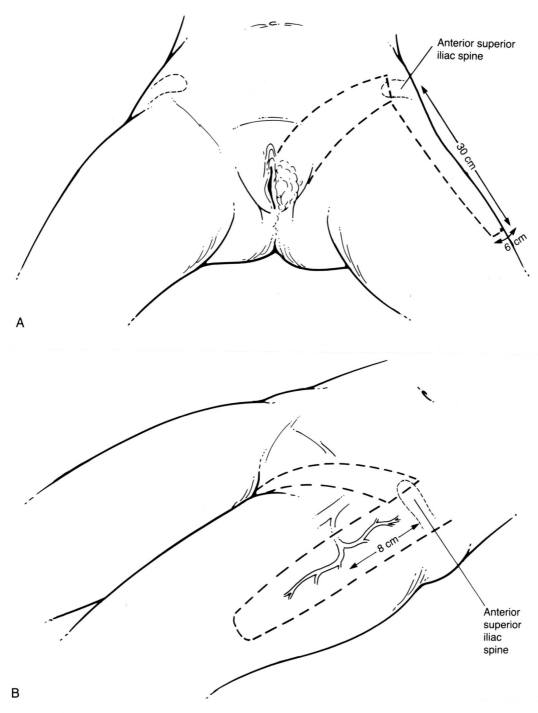

A

B

Figure 17-2. *A,* An overview of the flap, showing a potential use in gynecologic oncology. The flap can be used for repair of defects of the groin, lower abdomen, vulva, and perineum. The illustration shows a flap 30 cm in length (as measured from the anterior superior iliac spine) and 6 cm in width. *B,* The blood supply to the tensor fascia lata is derived from branches of the lateral femoral circumflex artery. The blood supply enters the flap 8 cm (range 6 to 10 cm) distal to the anterior superior iliac spine.

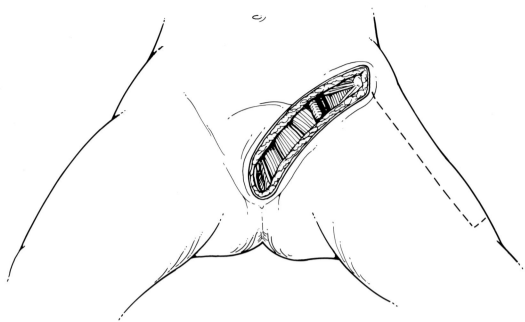

Figure 17-3. An example illustrating a radical resection of the groin contents and anterior vulva. The flap is outlined on the patient's lateral thigh. The anterior border extends from the anterior superior iliac spine to the lateral condyle of the knee. The posterior border of the flap corresponds to the greater trochanter. The distal border of the flap can extend to within 5 to 8 cm of the knee.

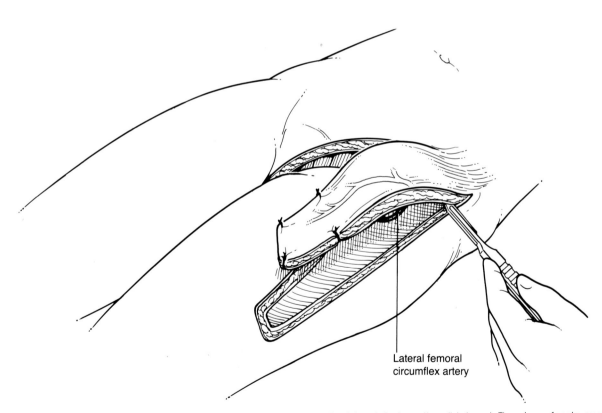

Lateral femoral
circumflex artery

Figure 17-4. The flap is being transected. The flap is initially elevated subfascially from the distal end. The deep fascia must be included with the flap to avoid disruption of the perforating vessels to the skin of the flap. The fascia may be temporarily sutured with 3-0 polyglycolic acid to the skin and subcutaneous tissues during flap transection. Care should be taken not to disrupt the arterial supply, which enters the flap 6 to 10 cm from the anterior superior iliac spine. The flap should be dissected superiorly far enough to allow adequate rotation.

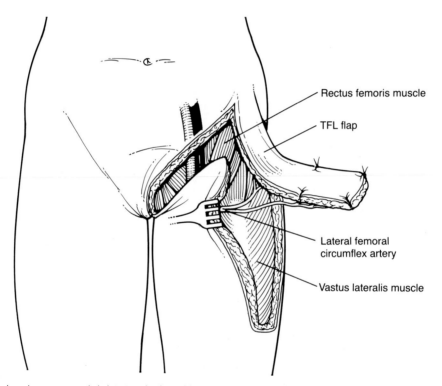

Rectus femoris muscle

TFL flap

Lateral femoral
circumflex artery

Vastus lateralis muscle

Figure 17–5. The flap has been completely resected and is now ready to be rotated into the anterior vulva and groin defect. Alternatively, the flap may be tunneled as indicated by the resection defect. If the flap is tunneled, the portion that lies underneath the skin bridge should be de-epithelialized.

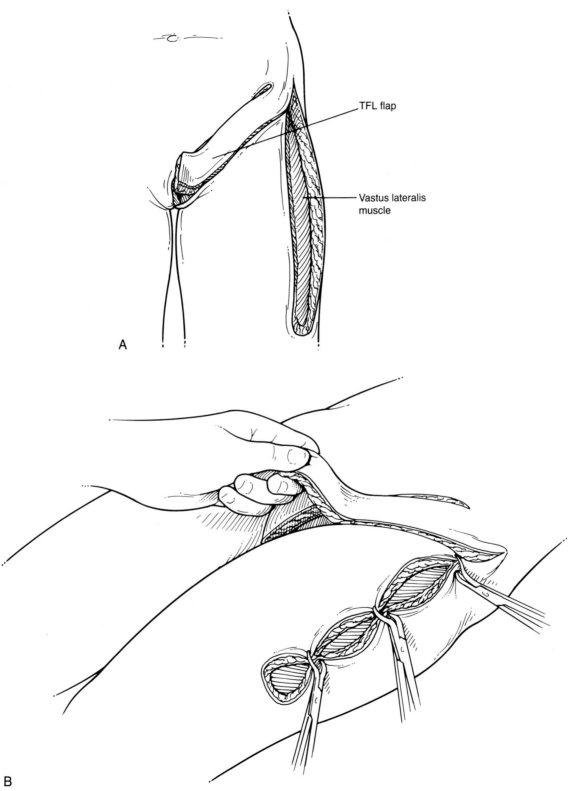

A

TFL flap

Vastus lateralis muscle

B

Figure 17–6. *A* and *B,* The flap has been rotated into the groin, and preparations are made to close the lateral thigh defect. The donor defect should not be closed if significant tension is present. It may be subsequently closed by secondary skin grafting.

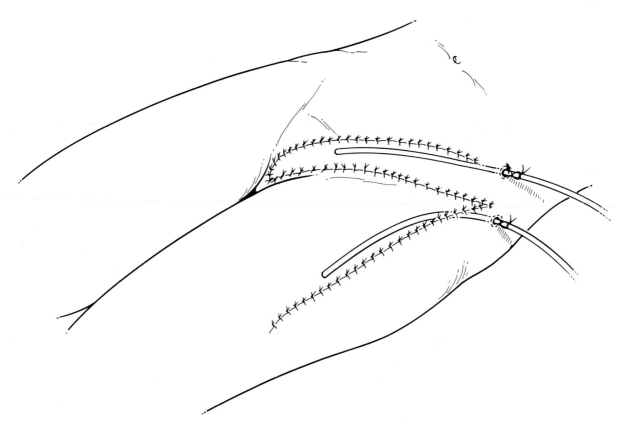

Figure 17–7. The flap has been sutured in place, and the thigh defect has been closed. Subcutaneous drains should be placed underneath the flap and in the thigh defect for drainage.

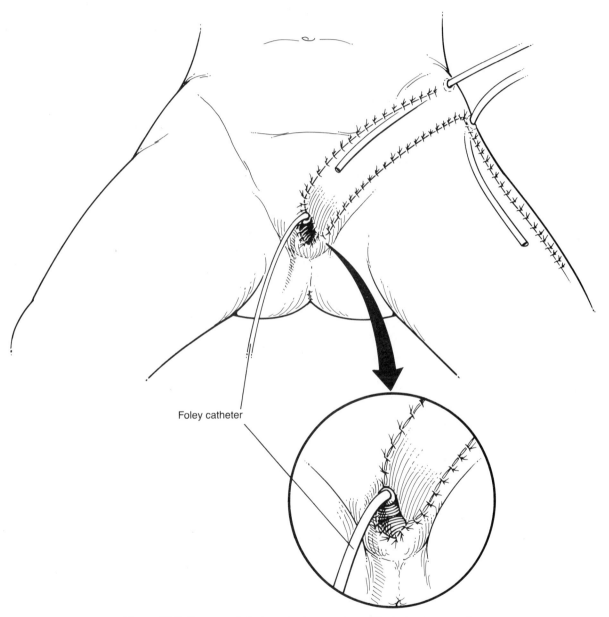

Foley catheter

Figure 17–8. The completed surgical procedure with drain placements.

CONCLUDING COMMENTS

The flap should not be placed on tension when suturing it into the operative site. Any tension may result in increased risk for flap necrosis. Drains should be placed beneath the flap donor site and also under the flap. The drains may be removed when drainage has decreased to less than 25 ml per 24 hours.

Patients undergoing this procedure may have numbness and may experience some difficulty with ambulation because of the area of the flap donor site. Patients should start physical therapy with muscular retraining as soon as feasible. Care should be taken when measuring the area of defect so that adequate length of the flap is taken to ensure that the defect is covered, and the flap is placed without tension. Closure of the flap donor site usually can be accomplished primarily. If necessary, owing to extreme tension, the flap donor site may be left open to granulate in. This area can be covered with secondary skin grafting at a later date.

REFERENCES

1. Bassett A: Traitement chirurgical operatoire de l'epithelioma primitif du clitoris: indications-techniques-résultats. Rev Chir 46:546, 1912.
2. Chafe W, Fowler WC, Walton LA, Currie JL: Radical vulvectomy with use of tensor fascia lata myocutaneous flap. Am J Obstet Gynecol 145:207–213, 1983.
3. Goldberg MI, Rothfleisch S: The tensor fascia lata myocutaneous flap in gynecologic oncology. Gynecol Oncol 12:41–50, 1981.
4. Hacker NF, Leuchter RS, Berek JS, et al: Radical vulvectomy and bilateral inguinal lymphadenectomy through separate groin incisions. Obstet Gynecol 58:574–579, 1981.
5. Knapstein PG, Friedberg V: Reconstructive operations of the vulva and vagina. In Knapstein PG, Friedberg V, Sevin B-U (eds): Reconstructive Surgery in Gynecology. Thieme, New York, 1990, pp 11–70.
6. Nahai F, Hill LH, Hester TR: Experiences with the tensor fascia lata flap. Plast Reconstr Surg 63:788–799, 1979.
7. Taussig F: Primary cancer of the vulva, vagina, and female urethra, five year results. Surg Gynecol Obstet 60:447, 1935.
8. Wangensteen OH: Repair of recurrent and difficult hernias and other large defects of the abdominal wall employing the iliotibial tract of fascia lata as a pedicled flap. Surg Gynecol Obstet 59:766–780, 1934.
9. Way S: The anatomy of the lymphatic drainage of the vulva and its influence on the radical operation for carcinoma. Ann R Coll Surg Engl 3:187, 1948.

18

Alternate Reconstructive Techniques for Repair of Large Vulvar and Vaginal Defects

Laurel A. King, M.D.

THE GLUTEAL THIGH FLAP

The development of reconstructive surgical techniques has facilitated recovery and lessened complications in patients who have undergone radical extirpative procedures for cancers of the female genital tract. The extended gluteal thigh flap, initially described by Hurwitz in 1980, is one such technique. The flap was initially used for reconstruction of complex pelvic wounds but also has found wide use in gynecologic oncology. The flap has been described for reconstruction after radical vulvectomy and for vaginal reconstruction after radical operative procedures. This flap is versatile and can be used to reconstruct large tissue defects of the perineum, vulva, vagina, and sacrum. It has also been used for reconstruction after radiation necrosis.

The flap is based on blood supply from the inferior gluteal artery. The inferior gluteal artery supplies the caudal portion of the gluteus maximus muscle. It then continues as a cutaneous vessel to the mid posterior portion of the thigh. The flap is usually no more than 12 cm wide and may extend lengthwise as far as the popliteal fossa. The donor site is usually easily closed primarily. The flap can be performed with the patient in the prone position or in the dorsal lithotomy position. In the dorsal lithotomy position, the gluteus maximus muscle overlies the ischial tuberosity, which is an important anatomic landmark. The inferior gluteal artery enters the flap medial to the ischial tuberosity. The posterior cutaneous nerve of the thigh also innervates the flap and, if included with the flap, allows the flap to be sensate. Formation of this flap, however, results in loss of sensation and numbness in the posterior thigh. The flap can be directly transposed into a surgical defect or tunneled. It can also be raised as an island flap and tunneled to the operative site. Use of this flap has been associated with very little morbidity.

Preoperative Management

The patient should receive prophylactic antibiotics. The procedure may be done in the dorsal lithotomy position. If so, the patient must be in a position that provides maximum flexion of the hips to allow identification of the surgical landmarks. If the flap is tunneled, the portion of the flap that goes underneath the skin tunnel must be de-epithelialized.

Potential Problem Areas

To allow adequate mobilization of the flap, the gluteus maximus muscle must be partially transected. Care must be taken not to transect the muscle beyond the posterior skin incision. This flap cannot be done in patients who have undergone prior hypogastric artery ligation, as in total pelvic exenteration. If this flap is planned for vaginal reconstruction at the time of pelvic exenteration, the hypogastric artery must not be ligated. Additionally, care should be taken during flap elevation not to disrupt the muscle and deep fascia away from the skin and subcutaneous tissues of the flap, in order to avoid compromise of the blood supply to the distal portion of the flap. The posterior cutaneous nerve courses posterior to the deep fascia of the thigh, and if it is included with the flap, the flap will be sensate. However, there may be resultant numbness in the posterior thigh area. The nerve does not have to be included with the flap if a sensate flap is not desired. Care must also be taken to allow adequate flap length to cover the surgical defect without tension. If the wound is closed with tension, flap necrosis may result. The donor site is usually closed primarily. If necessary, the donor site area may be left open to granulate and closed with skin grafting at a later time. Additionally, an attempt should be made to keep the point of rotation of the flap below the ischial tuberosity, in order to ensure adequate blood supply to the flap.

THE GLUTEAL THIGH FLAP

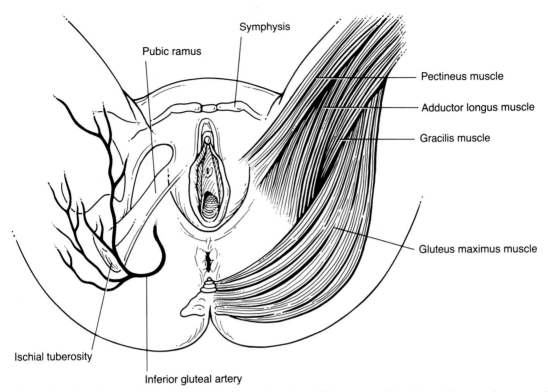

Figure 18–1. Overview of anatomy of the gluteal thigh flap. In the dorsal lithotomy position, the gluteus maximus muscle overlies the ischial tuberosity. The flap is centered on the posterior aspect of the thigh midway between the ischial tuberosity and the greater trochanter. The inferior gluteal artery is the basis of the blood supply to the flap. The inferior gluteal artery supplies the distal half of the gluteus maximus muscle and skin and then continues beyond the caudal edge of the muscle as a direct cutaneous posterior thigh vessel. The inferior gluteal artery enters the flap just medial to the ischial tuberosity. The posterior cutaneous nerve of the thigh runs below the deep fascia of the thigh parallel to the inferior gluteal artery.

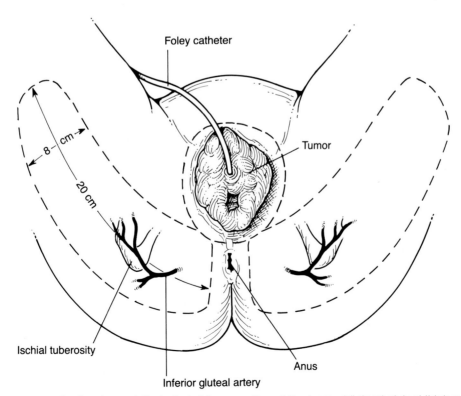

Figure 18–2. A large recurrent vulvar tumor is illustrated. After resection of the tumor, bilateral gluteal thigh myocutaneous flaps are planned. The flap can be as large as 12 cm in width and 32 cm in length. It is important to note the anatomic relation of the gluteal thigh flap to the ischial tuberosity.

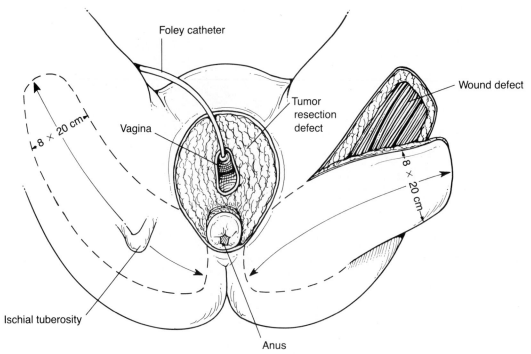

Figure 18–3. The surgical defect remaining after radical resection of the tumor is shown. The left gluteal thigh flap is resected. The resection should begin at the superior and lateral end of the flap and proceed medially.

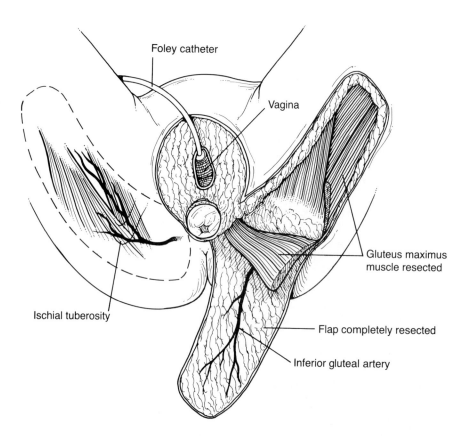

Figure 18–4. The gluteus maximus muscle must be partially transected to allow complete mobilization of the flap. The muscle can be partially transected with electrocautery. The gluteus maximus muscle is transected close to the base of the flap. The muscle must not be transected below the posterior skin incision. This procedure should not be performed in patients who have undergone prior hypogastric artery ligation. The skin and subcutaneous tissues (and, posteriorly, the gluteus maximus muscle) may be temporarily sutured with 3-0 polyglycolic acid to prevent flap disruption.

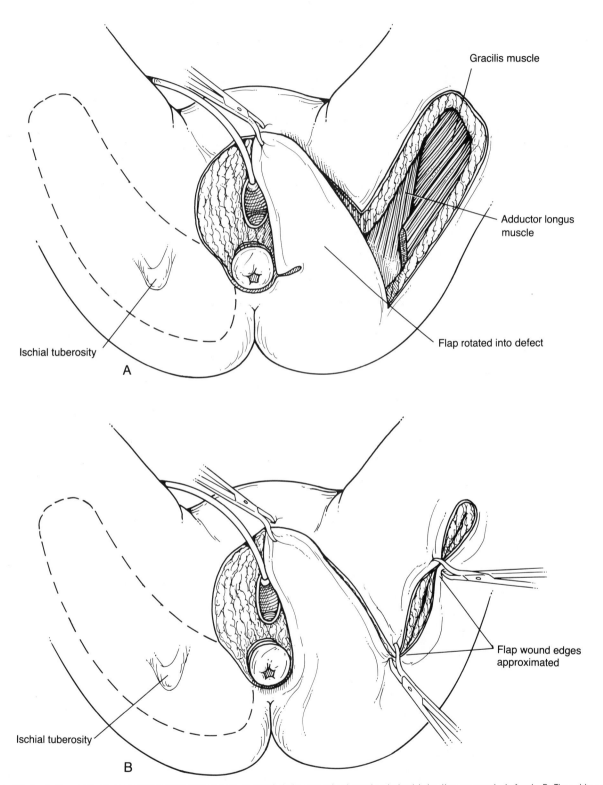

Figure 18–5. *A,* The left gluteal thigh flap has been completely resected and rotated into the wound defect. *B,* The skin and subcutaneous tissues are undermined over the thigh musculature and are then approximated for primary closure.

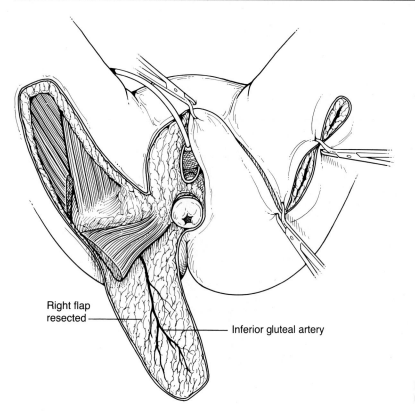

Right flap
resected

Inferior gluteal artery

Figure 18–6. The right gluteal thigh flap has been resected.

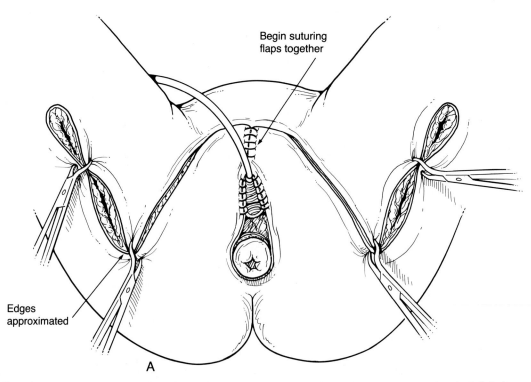

Begin suturing
flaps together

Edges
approximated

A

Figure 18–7. *A,* Both flaps have been placed into the surgical defect and the donor site approximated. Suturing of the wound has begun, using 3-0 polyglycolic acid sutures. The vagina, perineum, and anal and superior labial sutures are placed initially. *B,* The wound has been further sutured with closure of the donor site defects. Closed suction drainage should be used for the wound defects. *C,* Completion of the wound suturing, with the anus being sutured to the medial portions of the flap. Drains may be placed under the flap and brought out through a separate incision as well.

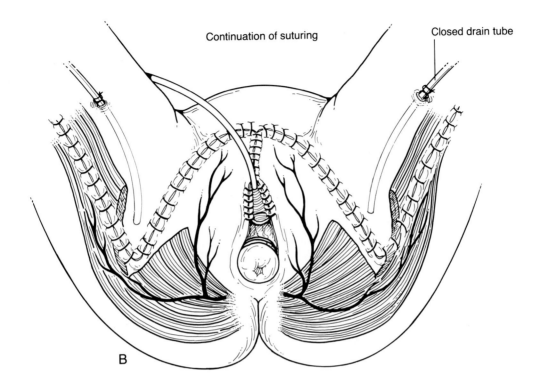

B

Continuation of suturing

Closed drain tube

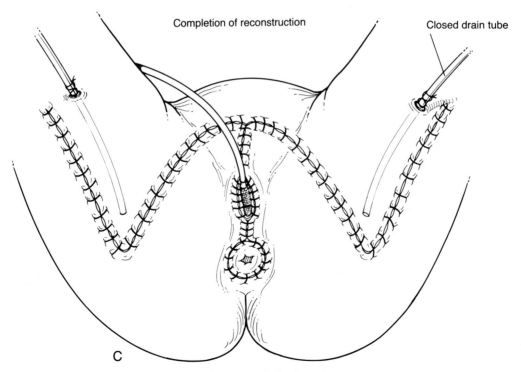

C

Completion of reconstruction

Closed drain tube

Figure 18–7 *Continued*

Concluding Comments

Closed suction drainage should be used in the donor bed site if it is closed primarily.

THE FASCIO-CUTANEOUS PUDENDAL-THIGH FLAP

The first fascio-cutaneous flap was described by Ponten in 1980. The fascio-cutaneous system of blood supply to the skin consists of blood vessels that reach the skin by passing along the fascial septa between adjacent muscle bellies and fan out at the level of the deep fascia to form a plexus from which blood reaches the skin. Wee and associates first described a pudendal-thigh flap that was used for vaginal reconstruction in 1989. Wee and Joseph described the use of this flap for vaginal reconstruction after total pelvic exenteration and for use in congenital vaginal agenesis.

This flap is unique in that it is easy to perform, has a very reliable blood supply, and is sensate. No stents or dilators are needed when a sensate flap is used to create a neovagina. The donor scars, which are centered on the thigh crease and groin, are well hidden when healing is complete.

This flap is useful for repair of vulvovaginal lesions after radical tumor resection, or after débridement of ulcers from radiation necrosis. It can be used either unilaterally or bilaterally. An additional advantage is that the flap is not bulky, as is often seen with myocutaneous flaps.

Preoperative Patient Preparation

The patient should receive prophylactic antibiotics prior to the proposed procedure. The flap is centered on the skin crease, which is (usually) lateral to the hair-bearing area of the vulva. The usual skin prep and shave or clip should be performed prior to starting the surgical case.

Potential Problem Areas

The flap is very reliable and easy to perform. However, the flap can only rotate through a 70-degree arc. This is usually satisfactory for neovagina formation and repair of defects of the vagina, posterior vulva, and perineal area. If the deep fascia over the aductor muscles is transected at the level of the vaginal introitus, the blood supply to the flap will be destroyed. If a bulky flap is necessary to repair large defects of the pelvis or for creation of a neovagina, then the fascio-cutaneous flap would not be the most appropriate procedure. A myocutaneous flap (i.e., gracilis) would be bulkier and might better serve the purpose.

THE FASCIO-CUTANEOUS PUDENDAL-THIGH FLAP

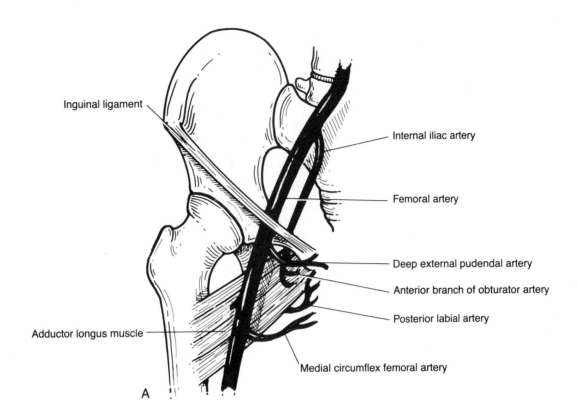

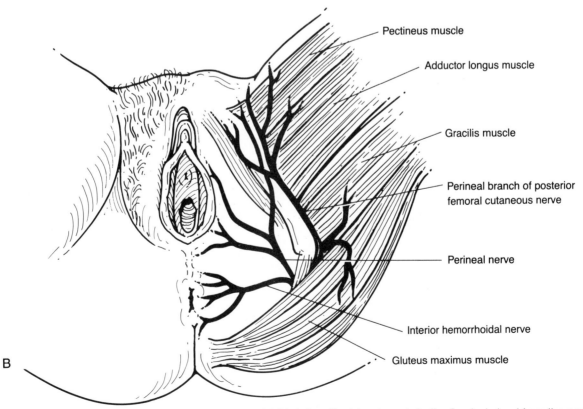

Figure 18–8. *A* and *B*, Overview of anatomy of the pudendal-thigh flap. The blood supply to the flap is derived from the posterior labial artery. The flap is well innervated from branches of the pudendal nerve and is sensate.

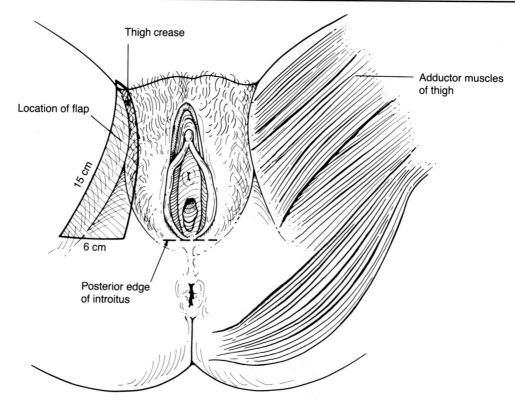

Figure 18–9. The location and anatomic landmarks of the pudendal-thigh flap. The flap is triangle shaped and centered in the thigh crease. The superior tip of the flap is located on the femoral triangle. The base of the flap is at the level of the posterior vaginal introitus. The flap may measure up to 6 cm in width at its base and 15 cm in length measured from the femoral triangle to the posterior introitus.

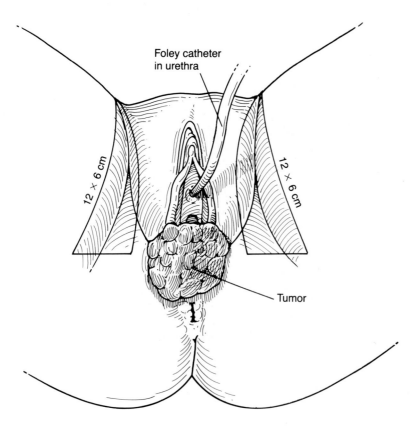

Figure 18–10. A lesion of the posterior vulva and perineum. Bilateral pudendal-thigh flaps are illustrated, each measuring 12 × 6 cm.

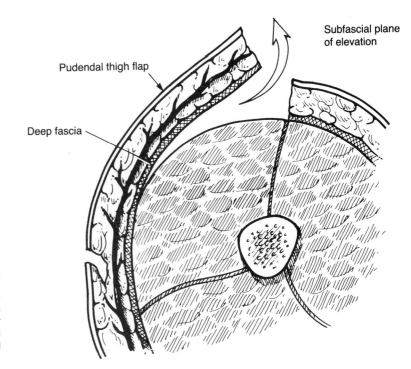

Figure 18–11. The subfascial plane of elevation. The deep fascia must be included with the flap. Care must be taken not to disrupt the fascia from its skin and subcutaneous tissue. The fascia may be loosely sutured to the skin and subcutaneous tissue during flap elevation with polyglycolic sutures. Elevation of the flap should begin superiorly, over the femoral triangle, and then extended inferiorly toward the posterior introitus. Although the skin and subcutaneous tissue are incised completely around the flap, the deep fascia is incised only to the level of the posterior vaginal introitus. If the fascia is cut at the level of the vaginal introitus, it will disrupt the blood supply to the flap.

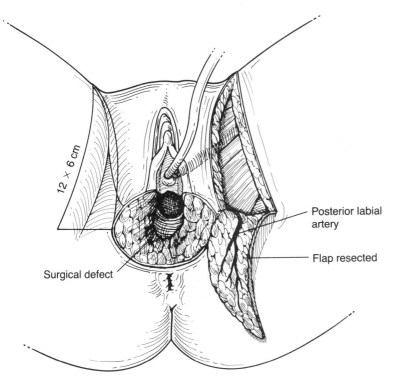

Figure 18–12. The flap has been resected completely on the patient's left side. A branch of the posterior labial artery is shown with the flap. The blood supply is easily identifiable on this flap.

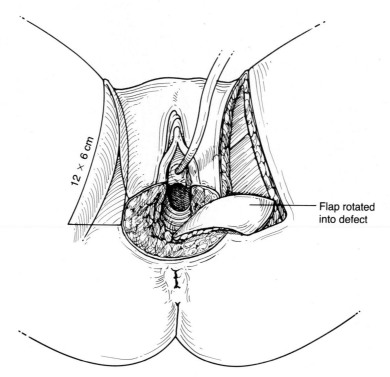

Figure 18–13. Note that the skin and subcutaneous tissue are completely incised on the flap, but the posterior fascia over the muscles at the level of the vaginal introitus is intact. The skin and subcutaneous tissue should be undermined suprafascially for about 4 cm at the base of the flap to allow for greater flap mobility. The flap can be rotated up to 70 degrees into the surgical defect. Likewise, the flap may be tunneled under a skin bridge. If the flap is tunneled, the portion of the flap that is under the skin bridge should be de-epithelialized.

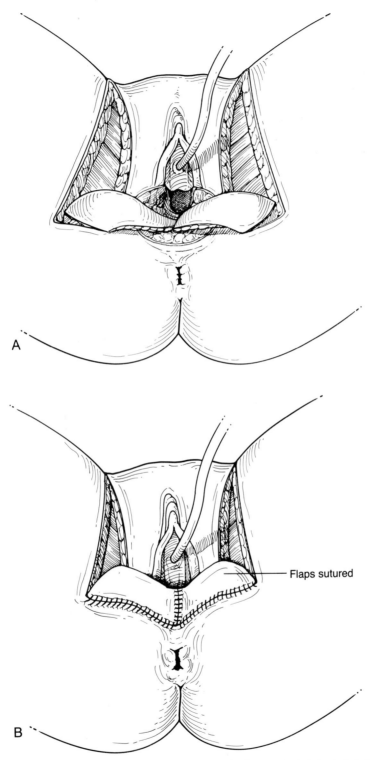

Figure 18–14. *A,* Bilateral pudendal-thigh flaps with rotation of the flaps into the surgical defect. *B,* Suturing of the flaps has begun to the perineum, vagina, and posterior vulva.

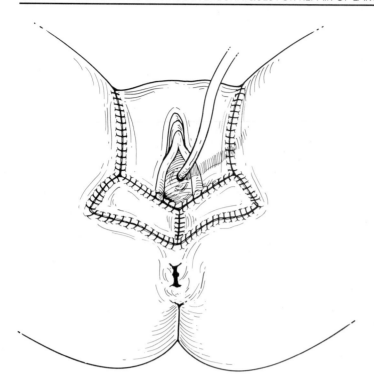

Figure 18–15. Completed suturing of the flaps to the vaginal wall and perineum, with closure of the surgical defect. Note that the flap donor site is centered over the thigh crease and the scar is hidden in the thigh crease when healed. Drains are usually not necessary.

REFERENCES

The Gluteal Thigh Flap

1. Achauer BM, Braly P, Berman ML, DiSaia PJ: Immediate vaginal reconstruction following resection for malignancy using the gluteal thigh flap. Gynecol Oncol 19:79–89, 1984.
2. Achauer BM, Turpin IM, Furnas DW: Gluteal thigh flap in reconstruction of complex pelvic wounds. Arch Surg 118:18–22, 1983.
3. Hurwitz DJ: Closure of a large defect of the pelvic cavity by an extended compound myocutaneous flap based on the inferior gluteal artery. Br J Plast Surg 33:256–261, 1980.
4. Knapstein PG, Friedberg V: Reconstructive operations of the vulva and vagina. In Knapstein PG, Friedberg V, Sevin B-U (eds): Reconstructive Surgery in Gynecology. Thieme, New York, 1990. pp 11–70.

The Fascio-Cutaneous Pudendal-Thigh Flap

1. Cormack GC, Lamberty BGH: A classification of fascio-cutaneous flaps according to their patterns of vascularization. Br J Plast Surg 37:80–87, 1984.
2. Ponten B: The fascio-cutaneous flap: Its use in soft tissue defects of the lower leg. Br J Plast Surg 34:215, 1981.
3. Wee JTK, Joseph VT: A new technique of vaginal reconstruction using neurovascular pudendal-thigh flaps: A preliminary report. Plast Reconstr Surg 83:701–709, 1989.

Index

Note: Page numbers in *italics* refer to illustrations; page numbers followed by *t* refer to tables. Boldface numbers refer to main discussions.

Abdominal incisions, and closures, **44–51**
  basic criteria for, 44
  midline types of, 44, *44*
  transverse types of, 44, *44*, *45*, *46*
Abdominal wall, anterior, arterial blood supply of, *45*
  muscle layers of, *109*
Abductor longus muscle, *38*
ACE inhibitors, 2, 16
Acquired immunodeficiency syndrome (AIDS), 4
Acute tubular necrosis, 19
Adductor brevis muscle, *235*
Adductor longus muscle, *232*, *234*, *235*
Adductor longus tendon, *233*
Adductor magnus muscle, *235*
Adnexa removal, in radical hysterectomy, *82*
AIDS (acquired immunodeficiency syndrome), 4
Albuterol, 17
A-lines, 5
Allen stirrups, *165*
Analgesia, patient-controlled, 19
Anal sphincter muscle, external, *215*
Angiotensin converting enzyme inhibitors, for perioperative period, 2, 16
Anovaginal fistula. *See* Rectovaginal fistula.
Anterior fascia, *160*, *161*
Anterior pelvic exenteration, *165–169*
  contraindications for, 164
  field of dissection for, *168*
  indications for, 164
  pathophysiologic changes from, 164
  potential problem areas in, 164–165
  treatment failure and, 164
Anterior rectus sheath, *110*
Anterior superior iliac spine, 27, *241*, *242*
Anterior thoracic artery, *45*
Anterior triangle, apex or crotch of, *7*, *10*
  localization of, *7*, *11*

Antibiotics, prophylactic use of, 6, 16, 16*t*, 17*t*
Anticoagulants, for deep vein thrombosis prophylaxis, 20
Antihypertensive medications, for perioperative period, 16
Anus, *210*
Aorta, anatomic relations of, *55*, *112*, *122*, *124*, *127*, *137*
  bifurcation of, *67*, *127*, *145*, *150*
  exposure of, *121*
Aortic lymph nodes, biopsies of, *68*. *See also* Para-aortic nodes, evaluation of.
Aortic stenosis, 2
Appendix, *185*
Arcuate line (semilunar line), *109*, *110*
Arcus tendineus, *144*
Argon beam coagulator, 88
Army/Navy retractor, *119*
Arterial blood gases, preoperative evaluation of, 5
Ascending colon, *186*
Ascites, 89
Asthma, 3
Atelectasis, 3

Babcock clamp, *99*
Beta-2–aerosols, perioperative use of, 17
Beta blockers, abrupt withdrawal of, 2, 16
  for thyrotoxic patient, 18
Bilateral rhomboid skin flaps, *229*
Biopsy, lymph node, *68*
Bladder, anatomic relations of, *67*, *69*, *95*, *142*, *148*, *168*, *177*
  after radical hysterectomy, *85*
  cross-sectional view of, *141*, *143*, *144*, *145*, *147*
  in relation to rectovaginal fistula, *219*
  in vesicocervical space development, *75*, *94*
  lateral view of, *90*, *92*, *93*
  pelvic spaces and, *70*

Bladder *(Continued)*
  with vesicouterine space, *173*
  involvement of, in advanced ovarian cancer, 88
  mobilization of, *166*
  operative injury of, 196
  separation of, from symphysis pubis, *143*
  with adherent ovarian cancer, 89
Blake drainage system, 29, 54, *118*, *124*
Bleeding diathesis, 5
Blood gases, arterial, preoperative evaluation of, 5
Blood pressure, preoperative assessment of, 3
Boari-Ockerblad method, for distal ureter injury repair, *205*, 206
Bovie, *119*
Bowel obstruction, from pelvic exenteration, 164
Bowel preparation, for continent urinary reservoir, 184
  potassium supplementation for, 19
  preoperative method for, 17, 18*t*
Breakaway introducer, for Groshong catheter placement, *20*, *21*
  for subclavian vein catheterization, *15*, *16*
Breast taping technique, for visualization of operative field, 12
Bronchospastic disease, perioperative therapy for, 3, 17
Bulbocavernosus muscle, anatomic relations of, *215*
  removal of, in radical vulvectomy, *40*

Calcium channel blockers, perioperative considerations for, 2, 16
Camper's fascia, 28, 29
Cancer. *See at specific anatomic site, e.g.,* Cervical cancer.
Cancer family syndrome, 4*t*

Cardiac failure, physical examination for, 2–3
Cardiac reserve, testing of, 3
Cardinal ligament(s), anatomic relations of, *94–95*, *141*, *146*
 cross-sectional view of, *70*, *71*
 division of, *103*, *167*, *175*
 transection of, in modified radical hysterectomy, *63*
Cardiovascular medications, for perioperative therapy, *16t*, 16–17
Cardiovascular system, disease of, perioperative therapy for, *16t*, 16–17, *17t*
 postoperative complications of, 16
 prophylactic antibiotics for, 16, *16t*
 preoperative evaluation of, 2–3
Carotid artery, catheterization of, 6
 palpation of, *7, 9*
Catheter. *See specific type, e.g.,* Malecot catheter.
Caval lymph nodes, biopsies of, *68*. *See also* Para-aortic nodes, evaluation of.
CBC (complete blood count), 4
Cecostomy drain, *192*, *194*
Cecostomy tube, *193*
Cecum, *186*
Central venous access, for long-term therapy, 20
 for pulmonary artery catheterization, 5
 general principles of, 5–6
 internal jugular vein for, anterior triangle approach in, 6, *7–11*
  complications of, 6, *9*
  seeker needle placement for, *8*
  surgical anatomy of, *7*
 preoperative planning for, 19
 Seldinger technique for, 6, *6*
 subclavian approach for, 6, *12–15*
 Trendelenburg position for, *12*
Cervical cancer, irradiated, total pelvic exenteration of. *See* Total pelvic exenteration.
 para-aortic node involvement in, 126
 radical hysterectomy for, 66
 staging procedures for, 108
Cervix, *63*, *143, 144, 145*
Cherney incision, *47, 55*
Chest x-ray, preoperative, 5
Chronic obstructive pulmonary disease (COPD), 3, 5, *9*
Cigarette use, history of, 3
Circumflex artery, deep, *45*
 lateral, *233*
 lateral femoral, *241, 243, 244*
 medial, *233*
 superficial, *214*
Circumflex iliac vein, *58*
Circumflex vein, deep, *55*
Clavicle, anatomic relations of, *7, 11, 13*
 head of, *7*
 middle third of, *7, 12*
Clitoris, *155*
Clonidine withdrawal, 16
Cloquet node, *38*
Closed drainage system, for obese patients, with midline incision, *51*
 for vesicovaginal fistula repair, *202*
Coagulation tests, 4–5
Colic artery, left, *185*
 middle, *170, 185, 186*
 right, *185, 186*
Colles fascia, incision of, *40*
Colon. *See also* Sigmoid colon.

Colon *(Continued)*
 anatomic relations of, *178, 185*
 ascending, *186*
 Heineke-Mikulicz reconfiguration for, *192*
 left, reflection of, *136–138*
 loop of, pulled through stoma, *172*
 right, *127*
  reflection of, *131–135*
 transverse, *171*
 vascular supply of, *185*
Colpocleisis, partial, Latzko technique for, *196–199*
Common iliac artery, *77, 112, 116, 121, 127, 145, 146, 150, 152, 153*
Common iliac vein, *55, 121, 127, 145, 146, 150, 152, 153*
Complete blood count (CBC), 4
Computed tomography (CT), for preoperative evaluation, 5
Congestive heart failure, 16, 19
Connective tissue syndromes, 5
Continent urinary reservoir, **184–194**
 colon reconfiguration for, *192*
 creation of continent mechanism for, *188–190*
 historical aspects of, 184
 ileal stoma site for, *193*
 indications for, 184
 intestinal segment, detubulization of, *187*
 irrigation of pouch, *194*
 management of, *194*
 potential problem areas for, 184
 preoperative preparation for, 184
 resection site for, *186*
 stoma for, *193*
 upper tract deterioration and, 184
 ureter transection for, *191*
Cooper's ligament, *56*
COPD (chronic obstructive pulmonary disease), 3, 5, *9*
Coronary angiography, 5
Coronary artery disease, 2, 5
Coumadin, for deep vein thrombosis prophylaxis, 20
Cribriform fascia, *29*
Cricothyroid membrane, *10, 11*
CT (computed tomography), for preoperative evaluation, 5
Cul-de-sac, *73*
CUSA, 88

Debulking, for advanced ovarian cancer, 88, *89–96*
Deep circumflex artery, *45*
Deep circumflex vein, *55*
Deep epigastric vessels, *45*
Deep external sphincter muscle, *214*
Deep femoral artery, *233*
Deep inferior epigastric artery, *45, 49, 50, 115*
Deep inferior epigastric vein, *49, 50, 115*
Deep uterosacral ligament, *146*
Deep vein thrombosis (DVT), prophylaxis for, 19–20
 risk factors for, 19
Deltopectoral groove, *12*
Demel-bladder splitting technique, *205*, 206
Diabetes, endocrine disorders and, 4
 insulin-dependent type of, 18

Diabetes *(Continued)*
 non–insulin-dependent type of, 18
 silent myocardial infarction risk and, 2
Diabetic ketoacidosis (DKA), 18
Dialysis, 19
Distal ureter injuries, repair of, **196–206**, *202–206*
 Boari-Ockerblad method for, *205*
 closure for, *206*
 Demel technique for, *205*
 incisions for, *203*
 pathophysiologic changes from, 196
 patient position for, *196*
 potential problem areas in, 196
 submucosal tunnel for, *204*
 sutures for, *205*
Diuretics, 2, 16
DKA (diabetic ketoacidosis), 18
Drainage, Blake system for, *29*, 54, *118, 124*
 closed system of, for obese patients, with midline incision, *51*
 for vesicovaginal fistula repair, *202*
 for radical vulvectomy, 34, *42*
 Jackson-Pratt system for, *29*, 54, *84, 85, 118, 124*
 of gastrostomy, *99*
Duodenum, *134, 135*
DVT (deep vein thrombosis), prophylaxis for, 19–20
 risk factors for, 19
Dyspnea, on exertion, 2, 3

ECG (electrocardiogram), 5
Edema, pulmonary, 16
Elderly, pulmonary function tests for, 5
Electrocardiogram (ECG), 5
Electrolyte abnormalities, 5
Endocrine system, preoperative evaluation of, 4
Endometrial cancer, para-aortic node evaluation for, 126
Endopelvic fascia, *217, 218*
End-stapling device, *105*
Epidural catheters, for narcotic analgesia, 19
Epigastric artery, deep inferior, *45, 49, 50, 115*
 superior, 45
Epigastric vein, deep inferior, *49, 50, 115*
Exercise stress tests, false-positives, in women, 5
Exterior oblique muscle, *36*
External anal sphincter muscle, *215*
External iliac artery, anatomic relations of, *45, 55, 58, 59, 67, 73, 90, 112, 116, 150, 151, 166*
 paravesical space and, *71*
 psoas muscle and, *57*
 incision over, *117*
 palpation of, *121*
External iliac vein, *55, 57, 58, 67, 71, 73, 121, 151, 166*
External inguinal ring, *38*
External oblique fascia, retraction of, *114*
External oblique muscle, anatomic relations of, *109*
 closure of, *118*
 incision of, *113*
 retraction of, *115*
 separation of, for stoma creation, *160, 161*

External oblique muscle *(Continued)*
  strap muscles and, *110*
External pudendal artery ligation, *37*
External sphincter muscle, dissection of,
    for rectovaginal fistula repair, *212*
  subcutaneous, *212*
  superficial, *212*
Extraperitoneal space, *117, 124*

Familial colonic polyposis, 4t
Fascia, anterior, *160, 161*
  Camper's, *28–29*
  cribriform, *29*
  endopelvic, *217, 218*
  external oblique, *114*
  posterior, *160, 161*
  psoas, *205*
  rectus, *47, 119*
  transverse, *109*, 110
Fascia lata, *36*
Femoral artery, anatomic relations of, *38,
    233, 241*
  coverage of, by transplanted sartorius
      muscle, *39*
Femoral sheath, *36*
Femoral vein, anatomic relations of, *38,
    241*
  coverage of, by transplanted sartorius
      muscle, *39*
  dissection of, for radical vulvectomy, *37*
FIGO TNM classification, 34
Fistulas, 5
  rectovaginal. *See* Rectovaginal fistula.
  vesicovaginal. *See* Vesicovaginal fistu-
      las.
Fluid status, perioperative management
    of, 18–19
Foley catheter, *206, 224*

Gallbladder, *131, 135*
Gardner's syndrome, 4t
Gastroepiploic arteries, *98, 178*
Gastroepiploic vein, *98*
Gastrointestinal anastomosis stapler
    (GIA), *149, 170, 220*
Gastrointestinal system, autosomal
    dominant syndromes of, 4t
  diseases of, preoperative evaluation for,
      3–4
  familial syndromes of, 4t
  perioperative therapy for, 17, 18t
  symptoms of, 5
Gastrostomy, *96–100*
Gastrostomy tube, distal end of, *100*
Genitofemoral nerve, *57, 58, 117*
GIA (gastrointestinal anastomosis
    stapler), *149, 170, 220*
Gibson incision, modified version of, for
    para-aortic node exposure, *111–113*
Glucocorticoids, 18
Gluteal artery, inferior, *250*
Gluteal thigh flap, anatomy of, *250*
  historical development of, 250
  innervation of, 250
  patient position for, 250
  potential problem areas for, 250
  preoperative management of, 250
Gluteus maximus muscle, blood supply of,
    250
Goblet cells, 3

Gracilis muscle, anatomic relations of,
    232
  cutaneous anatomy of, *233*
  identification of, distal approach for,
      234
    proximal approach for, *234*
Gracilis myocutaneous flap, anterior
    border, cutting of, *235*
  closure of, *237*
  drainage for, *237*
  for vaginal reconstruction, 232
  identification of muscle for, *234*
  potential problem areas of, 232
  sectioning of proximal insertion fascia
      for, *236*
  vascular pedicles and, *233*
Graves' disease, 4
Groin incision, for excisional biopsy of
    vulva, *27*
Grooved director, *159*
Groshong catheter placement, final
    closure for, *22*
  Groshong tunneler for, *21, 22*
  protective hub for, *22*
  technique for, *20–22*
Groshong tunneler, for Groshong catheter
    placement, *21, 22*
Guaiac stool test, 5
Guide wire, for subclavian vein
    catheterization, *15, 16*
  placement of, *14*
  J-type, *14, 20*

Hematocrit, 19
Hemorrhoidal vessels, superior, *149*
Hemothorax, 6
Heparin, for deep vein thrombosis
    prophylaxis, 20
Hepatic flexure, *186*
Hepatitis, 4
Hepatosplenomegaly, 4
Hyperalimentation, 89, 208
Hyperlipidemia, 2
Hypertension, perioperative morbidity
    and, 2
  renal insufficiency and, 4
Hypertensive crisis, in postoperative
    period, 17
Hyperthyroidism, 4
Hypoadrenalism, 4
Hypogastric artery, anatomic relations of,
    55, 59, 77, 146, 147, 150
  anterior division of, *151*
  obliterated, *71, 144*
Hypogastric vein, *146*
Hypotension, prolonged, 19
Hypothyroidism, 4, 17
Hysterectomy, modified radical. *See*
    Modified radical hysterectomy.
  radical. *See* Radical hysterectomy.
  reverse method for, *92, 101–105*
  vaginal, vesicovaginal fistulas and, 196

IDDM (insulin-dependent diabetes
    mellitus), 18
Ileal artery, *185, 186*
Ileal conduit, 184
Ileal loop, isolation of, *156*
Ileocecal valve, anatomic relations of,
    187, 193

Ileocecal valve *(Continued)*
  plication of, *190*
Ileocolic artery, *185, 186*
Ileus, intestinal, 89
Iliac artery, *115*
  external. *See* External iliac artery.
  internal, *112, 116*
Iliac crest, *118*
Iliac spine, anatomic relations of, *35*
  anterior superior, *27, 241, 242*
Iliac vein, circumflex, *58*
  external, *55, 57–58, 67, 71, 73, 121,
      151,* 166
Imaging, for preoperative evaluation, 5
Incision(s), abdominal. *See* Abdominal
    incisions.
  circular, for rectovaginal fistula repair,
      217
  middle. *See* Midline incision(s).
  modified Gibson, for para-aortic node
      exposure, *111–113*
  of groin, for excisional biopsy of vulva,
      27
  Schuchardt's, for vesicovaginal fistula
      repair, *197*
  vertical, bladder, for distal ureter in-
      jury repair, *203–206*
Indiana pouch, 165, *188*
Inferior gluteal artery, 250
Inferior mesenteric artery, *122, 123, 128,
    129, 137, 149, 185*
Inferior vena cava, *112*
Infundibulopelvic ligament, *68, 142*
Infundibulum ligament, *73*
Inguinal ligament, *27, 28, 36, 39*
Inguinal ring, external, *38*
Insulin therapy, perioperative, 18
Insulin-dependent diabetes mellitus
    (IDDM), 18
Internal iliac artery, *112, 116*
Internal jugular vein, anatomic relations
    of, *7, 10*
  in subclavian approach, *13*
  catheterization of, for long-dwelling
      catheter, 20
  central venous access of, using anterior
      triangle approach, 6, *7–11*
Internal oblique muscle, *109, 110, 114,
    118*
Intestinal ileus, 89
Intravenous pyelography (IVP), 5, 194
Introducer. *See* Breakaway introducer;
    Splitting introducer.
Ischiocavernosus muscle, anatomic
    relations of, *41, 154*
  removal of, in radical vulvectomy, *40*
Ischiorectal fat, *152, 153, 154*
IVP (intravenous pyelography), 5, 194

J guide wire, for Groshong catheter
    placement, *20*
  for subclavian vein catheterization, *14*
J ureteral catheter, *171*
Jack-knife position, *66*
Jackson-Pratt drainage system, *29*, 54,
    118, 124
  for radical hysterectomy, *84, 85*
Jejunal artery, *185, 186*
J-shaped incision, for para-aortic node
    exposure, *111–113*
Jugular vein, internal. *See* Internal
    jugular vein.

Juvenile polyposis, *4t*

Kidney, anatomic relations of, *131, 132, 135, 137*
  insufficiency of, perioperative therapy for, 19
    preoperative evaluation of, 4
  perioperative fluid maintenance and, 18–19
  physical examination of, 4
Kocher clamps, *102*
Kock continent ileostomy, as urinary reservoir, 184

Labial fat pad graft, for vesicovaginal fistula repair, *201–202*
Labia majora, *40*
Labia minora, *40*
Laboratory testing, preoperative, 4–5
Lateral circumflex artery, *233*
Lateral femoral circumflex artery, *241, 243, 244*
Latzko partial colpocleisis, operative technique for, *197–199*
  patient position for, *196*
Lawson position, *196*
Left colic artery, *185*
Left ventricular failure, 2–3
Leiomyomata, 5
Levator ani muscle, anatomic relations of, *83, 144*
  in rectovaginal fistula repair, *214, 215*
  in total pelvic exenteration, *151, 152, 153, 154*
  in perineal phase of posterior pelvic exenteration, *180*
Lifeport catheter placement. *See* Groshong catheter placement.
Linea alba, *109, 119*
Lithotomy position, modified, for anterior pelvic exenteration, *165*
Liver, alcoholic disease of, 3
  anatomic relations of, *131*
Loop diuretics, 2, 3
Lymphadenectomy, for radical hysterectomy, beginning of, *83*
  for total pelvic exenteration, *150*
Lymphangiography, 5
Lymph nodes, aortic, *68*
  bilateral groin dissection of, 26
  caval, *68*
    completed view of, *39*
    deep limit of, *40*
    packing for, *40*
    upper limit for, *38*
  extraperitoneal pelvic, dissection of, **54–64**
  para-aortic. *See* Para-aortic nodes.
  pelvic, dissection of, indications for, *38*
Lymphocyst, 108

Magnetic resonance imaging (MRI), 140
Major pedicle, *233*
Malecot catheter, *99, 100*
Martius bulbocavernosus flap, for vesicovaginal fistula repair, *201–202*
Mattress suture, modified, *226*
Maylard incision, closure of, *46*

Maylard incision *(Continued)*
  for modified radical hysterectomy, *55*
  operative technique for, *44, 45, 46*
Mechanical ventilation, in perioperative period, 17
Medial circumflex artery, *233*
Medial condyle of knee, *233*
Mesenteric artery, inferior, *122–123, 128–129, 137, 149, 185*
  superior, *185, 186*
Metaproterenol, 3, 17
Metzenbaum scissors, *225*
Miami pouch type urinary diversion, 165, *186*
Middle colic artery, *170, 185, 186*
Middle sacral vessels, *145, 147, 150, 151, 153*
Midline incision(s), advantages of, 44
  eviscerations of, 44
  for debulking of ovarian cancer, 88
  for direct transperitoneal approach to para-aortic nodes, *127*
  for modified radical hysterectomy, *55*
  for obese patients, *50–51*
    closure of, *51*
  for omentectomy, *96*
  for reflection of left colon, *136*
  for reflection of right colon, *131*
  operative technique for, 44, *44*
  radiation therapy and, 108
Minor vascular pedicles, *233*
Mitral stenosis, 2
Modified Gibson incision, for para-aortic node exposure, *111–113*
Modified radical hysterectomy,
    advantages of, 54
  classification of, 54
  exposure of pelvic space for, *56*
  historical aspects of, 54
  incision for, *55*
  operative technique for, *57–64*
  pathophysiologic changes from, 54
  potential problem areas in, 54
  sectioning of round ligament for, *56*
  with extraperitoneal pelvic lymph node dissection, **54–64**
MRI (magnetic resonance imaging), 140
Muscle relaxants, 2
Musculophrenic artery, *45*
Mushroom catheter, *99, 100*
Myocardial infarction, in postoperative period, 16
  risk, preoperative history and, 2
Myocutaneous flaps. *See also* Gracilis myocutaneous flap.
  for pelvic exenteration, 164

Nasogastric suctioning, potassium supplementation for, 19
Neck, anterior triangle of. *See* Anterior triangle.
Neck vein distention, 2
Neovaginal pouch, creation of, *236*
NIDDM (non–insulin-dependent diabetes mellitus), 18
Nitroglycerin, 16
Nitroprusside, 16
Non–insulin-dependent diabetes mellitus (NIDDM), 18
Non-polyposis syndrome, *4t*

Obesity, cricothyroid membrane in, localization of, *10*
  definition of, 4
  lymph node staging and, 126
  midline abdominal incision for, *50–51*
  sternocleidomastoid muscle junction and, *8*
Oblique muscle, exterior, *36*
  external. *See* External oblique muscle.
  internal, *109, 110, 114, 118*
Obturator internus muscle, *144*
Obturator nerve, anatomic relations of, *55, 56, 58, 83, 84, 166*
  in total pelvic exenteration, *150, 151, 152, 153*
Obturator vessels, *144, 150*
Oliguria, 18–19
Omentectomy, *96–100*
  spleen trauma and, 88
Omentum, anatomic relations of, *96, 169, 221*
  interposition of, between vagina and rectum, *220*
  mobilization of, *170*
  posterior attachment of, division of, *178*
  suturing of, to psoas muscle, *169, 172*
  wrapping of, around rectal stump anastomosis, *179*
Orthopenia, history of, 2
Ovarian artery, cutting of, *94*
Ovarian cancer, debulking for, *89–96*
  extent of, *97*
  optimal extent of, 88
  dissection plane for, 88, *93*
  surgical management of, **88–105**
    optimal extent of excision for, 88
    pathophysiologic changes from, 88–89
    potential complications of, 88
Ovarian pedicle, *173*
Ovarian vessels, anatomic relations of, *59, 69, 122, 142, 145, 146, 147*
  in reflection of right colon, *132*
  ureter and, *137*
  with ureter, *128, 130*
  skeletonization and division of, *92*
Ovaries, mobilization of, *92*

PAC. *See* Pulmonary artery catheters (PAC).
Pain management, postoperative, 19
Para-aortic nodes, evaluation of, in cervical cancer, 126
  in endometrial cancer, 126
  indications for, 126
  extraperitoneal approaches to, **108–124**
    J-shaped incision for, *111–113*
    potential problem areas for, 108
    right-sided approach for, *111*
  removal of, *117, 123*
  transperitoneal approach to, **126–138**
    direct method of, 126, *127–130*
    indications for, 126
    pathophysiology for, 126
    potential problem areas in, 126
    reflection of left colon in, *136–138*
    reflection of right colon in, *131–135*
Paracolic gutter, left, *136*
  right, *131*
Parametrium, anatomic relations of, *71, 72, 73, 74, 75, 78, 101, 147*
  clamping and division of, *167*

Parametrium (Continued)
  dissection of, for radical hysterectomy,
    79
  removal of, in radical hysterectomy, 82
Pararectal fossa, 147, 148
Pararectal space, anatomic relations of,
    73, 74, 76, 77, 78
  cross-sectional view of, 72, 101, 141
  development of, 72
    for modified radical hysterectomy, 60
  dissection of, 91
  uniting of, with paravesical space, 80
Paravesical fossa, 147, 148
Paravesical space, anatomic relations of,
    72, 73, 75, 76, 78, 94
  cross-sectional view of, 71, 101, 141,
    144
  development of, 70
  dissection of, 91
  uniting of, with pararectal space, 80
Parietal peritoneum, 161
Partial thromboplastin test (PTT), 4
Patient-controlled analgesia (PCA), 19
Pectineus muscle, dissection of, for
    radical vulvectomy, 38
Pelvic exenteration, anterior. See
    Anterior pelvic exenteration.
  posterior. See Posterior pelvic exentera-
    tion.
  total. See Total pelvic exenteration.
  transverse colon conduit for, 170–172
Pelvic spaces. See also Retrorectal space.
  creation of, complete mobilization of
    pelvic structures and, 147
  development of, 70, 143
    in anterior pelvic exenteration, 165
  pararectal. See Pararectal space.
  paravesical. See Paravesical space.
  prevesical, 141, 143, 147
  Retzius, space of, 55, 144, 202. See also
    Paravesical space; Prevesical
    space.
Pelvic viscera, 151
Pelvis, blood vessels of, 55
Penrose drain, 193, 194
Periaortic node, 142
Perineal muscle, superficial transverse,
    41, 154
Perineal skin, closure of, in rectovaginal
    fistula repair, 216
Perineoplasty, for radical vulvectomy, 42
  for rectovaginal fistula repair, 214
Perioperative management, 2–23
  central line placement for. See Central
    venous access.
  fluid therapy for, 18–19
  for cardiovascular disease, 16t, 16–17,
    17t
  for endocrine system, 17–18
  for gastrointestinal system, 17, 18t
  for pulmonary disease, 17
  prophylactic antibiotics for, 6
Periosteum, anesthesia of, for central line
    placement, 13
Peripheral artery catheterization, 5
Peritoneum, anatomic relations of, 67,
    110, 114
    after radical hysterectomy, 85
  blunt dissection of, 115, 121
  opening of, to sigmoid mesentery, 173
  over common iliac vessels, opening of,
    67
  parietal, 161

Peritoneum (Continued)
  retraction of, medially and cephalad,
    120
  visceral, 142
Peutz-Jeghers syndrome, 4t
Pfannenstiel incision, 44
  conversion of, to Cherney incision, 47
PFT (pulmonary function tests), 3, 5
Physical examination, for cardiovascular
    disease, 2–3
  of gastrointestinal system, 3–4
  of pulmonary system, 3
  of thyroid gland, 4
Pneumonia, 3
Pneumothorax, 6, 9
Polyposis, juvenile, 4t
Posterior fascia, 160, 161
Posterior pelvic exenteration, 173–181
  cardinal ligament division for, 175
  completed, view of, 181
  contraindications for, 164
  indications for, 164
  pathophysiologic changes from, 164
  perineal phase of, 180
  potential problem areas in, 164–165
  presacral space development for, 174
  rectal pillars division for, 176
  rectal stump anastomosis for, 177
  supralevator type of, 177
  treatment failure and, 164
  uterine artery ligation for, 175
  uterosacral ligament division for, 174
Posterior rectus sheath, 109–110
Postmenopausal patients, chest pain
    history in, 2
Postoperative management plan, 2
Potassium iodide, saturated solution of,
    18
Potassium supplementation, for bowel
    preparation, 19
  for nasogastric suctioning, 19
Pouch-o-gram, 194
Poupart's ligament, 142, 150
Preoperative period, gastrointestinal
    disease evaluation in, 3–4
  history taking in, 2–4
  invasive monitoring in, 5, 6t
  laboratory testing in, 4–5
  physical examination in, 2–4
Preoperative plan, importance of, 2
Presacral space, development of, 174
Prevesical space, 141, 143, 147
Promontorium, 148, 149, 150
Propylthiouracil, 18
Protective hub, for Groshong catheter, 22
Prothrombin test, 4
Psoas fascia, 205
Psoas muscle, anatomic relations of, 112,
    115, 121
    with external iliac artery and vein,
      57
  with sutured omentum, 172
PTT (partial thromboplastin test), 4
Pubic tubercle, 27
Pudendal artery, external, ligation of, 37
Pulmonary artery catheters (PAC),
    central venous access for, 5
  for congestive heart failure, 19
  for renal insufficiency, 19
  indications for, 5, 6t
Pulmonary edema, 16
Pulmonary function tests (PFT), 3, 5
Pulmonary system, complications of, risk
    factors for, 3t

Pulmonary system (Continued)
  diseases of, perioperative therapy for,
    17
  preoperative evaluation for, 3
Pyramidalis muscles, fascia of, separation
    from, 47
  raphe between, sectioning of, 51
  suturing of, 50

Radiation therapy, midline incision and,
    108
Radical hysterectomy, classification of, 54
  closure of, 85
  completion of, 84
  drainage of, 84, 85
  lymphadenectomy in, beginning of, 83
  modified technique for. See Modified
    radical hysterectomy.
  operative technique for, adnexa re-
    moval in, 82
    application of right-angle clamps in,
      81
    parametria removal in, 82
    parametrium dissection in, 79
    rectovaginal space development in,
      74
    uniting of pararectal space with para-
      vesical space in, 80
    upper vagina removal in, 82
    uterosacral ligament clamping in, 76
    uterus removal in, 82
    vesicouterine space development in,
      75
  vesicovaginal fistulas and, 196
  with pelvic node dissection, **66–85**
    incision for, 67
    indications for, 66
    jack-knife position for, 66
    potential problem areas for, 66
    preoperative evaluation for, 66
    urinary system monitoring for, 66
Radical vulvectomy, 26, **34–42**
  adipose tissue dissection for, 36
  butterfly incision for, 41
  closed drainage system for, 42
  completed dissection for, 41
  incision for, 35
  inferior flap for, 35
    dissection of, 36
  inner incision for, 40
  operative technique for, 36–38
  outer incision for, 40
  pathophysiologic changes from, 34
  postoperative care for, 34
  potential risks of, 34
  superior flap for, 35
Rales, 2
Rectal mucosa, 217
Rectal muscularis, 217, 218
Rectal pillars, division of, 176
Rectal stump anastomosis, for posterior
    pelvic exenteration, 177
  omentum wrap for, 179
Rectosigmoid, anatomic relations of, 142,
    147, 149, 150
  reanastomosis of, 221
  resection of, gastrointestinal anastomo-
    sis stapler for, 220
Rectovaginal fistula, classification of, 208
  etiology of, 208
  high, classification of, 208
  location of, 219

Rectovaginal fistula *(Continued)*
  repair of, *219–221*
    low, classification of, 208
      repair of, *209–216*
    mid, classification of, 208
      repair of, *217–218*
  operative techniques for, 208
  postoperative care for, 208
  preoperative evaluation for, 208
  reinforcement stitch for, *213–214*
  repair of, by conversion to complete
      perineal tear, *209*
    closure for, *216*
      deeper layer of perineal, completion
          of, *214–215*
      potential risks in, 208
      superficial layer of perineal, comple-
          tion of, *215–216*
    sutures, holding power of, 208
Rectovaginal septum, dissection of, *165*
Rectovaginal space, anatomic relations of,
    77, 78
  cross-sectional view of, *74, 141*
  development of, *74*
    for modified radical hysterectomy, *60*
  rectovaginal fistulas and, *217, 219*
Rectum, anatomic relations of, *151, 152,*
    168, 169, 217
  cross-sectional view of, *141, 143, 144,*
    145, 146
    to rectovaginal fistula, *219*
  closure of, for rectovaginal fistula re-
      pair, *220*
    transverse, for rectovaginal fistula
      repair, *218*
  division of, *105*
  separation of, from vagina, *210, 219*
Rectus abdominis muscle, *109*
Rectus fascia, *119*
Rectus femoris muscle, *232, 241, 244*
Rectus muscle, anatomic relations of, *36,*
    45, 110, 119
  dissection of, from insertion at sym-
      physis, *49*
  fascia of, separation from, *47*
  suturing of, *50*
  transection of, *120*
Rectus sheath, anterior, *110*
  posterior, *109–110*
Renal insufficiency. *See* Kidney,
    insufficiency of.
Renal vein, *138*
Retroperitoneal dissection, for debulking
    of advanced ovarian cancer, 88
Retroperitoneum, direct surgical
    approach for, 126, *127–130*
  lateral surgical approach for, 126
Retrorectal space, anatomic relations of,
    147
  cross-sectional view of, *141, 145, 146*
  opening of, *145*
Retzius, space of. *See also* Paravesical
    space; Prevesical space.
  anatomic relations of, *55, 144, 202*
  development of, *48, 51, 166*
Reverse hysterectomy, *92, 101–105*
Rhomboid skin flaps, angles for, *227*
  bilateral, *229*
  closure of, *228*
  for defects for vulvar carcinoma exci-
      sion, 224
  operative technique for, *227–228*
  physiologic changes from, 224
  postoperative care for, 224

Rhomboid skin flaps *(Continued)*
  potential problem areas in, 224
Right colic artery, *185, 186*
Right colon, *127*
Round ligament, anatomic relations of,
    69, 143
  division of, *90*
  isolation, clamping, sectioning and tied
      extraperitoneal, *115*
  sectioning of, for modified radical hys-
      terectomy, *56*
    for radical vulvectomy, *38*
  stump of, *68, 142*

Sacral plexus, *155*
Sacral promontory, *145*
Sacral vessels, middle, *145, 147, 150, 151,*
    153
Sacrum, *155*
Saphenous vein, ligation and sectioning
    of, for radical vulvectomy, *37*
Sartorius muscle, anatomic relations of,
    28, 38, 232, 233, 234, 235, 241
  transplantation of, *39*
Saturated solution of potassium iodide
    (SSKI), 18
Scarpa triangle, apex of, *35*
SCD (sequential compression device), 19,
    20
Schuchardt's incision, for vesicovaginal
    fistula repair, *197*
Seeker needle placement, for internal
    jugular vein central line placement,
    8–9
  angle of, *9*
  common mistakes in, *9*
  correct placement of, *9*
  incorrect placement of, *9*
  for Seldinger technique, *6*
  for subclavian approach, *13*
Seldinger technique, 6, *6*
Semilunar line (arcuate line), *109, 110*
Semimembranosus muscle, *233, 234*
Semitendinosus muscle, *233, 234*
Sentinel nodes, removal of, *28–29*
Sequential compression device (SCD), 19,
    20
Sexual dysfunction, from total pelvic
    exenteration, 140
Sigmoid colon, anatomic relations of, *67,*
    74, 75, 76, 77, 89, 92, 93
  in posterior pelvic exenteration, *177*
  lateral view of, *90*
  conservative resection of, *149*
  disease of, debulking for, 88
  division of, at pelvic brim, *173*
  mesentery of, *149, 173*
  removal of, *104*
  sectioning of, *149*
  transection of, *105*
  and preparation of, in colostomy, *153*
Singley forceps, *123*
Skin bridge, *235*
Skin flaps, rhomboid. *See* Rhomboid skin
    flaps.
Smead-Jones closure, of midline incision,
    51
Sphincter ani, *154*
Sphincter muscle, deep external, *214*
  dissection of, *212*
  subcutaneous external, *214*
  superficial external, *214*

Sphincteroplasty, in rectovaginal fistula
    repair, *212–213*
Spleen, anatomic relations of, *96*
  laceration of, during omentectomy, *98*
Splenectomy, for debulking of advanced
    ovarian cancer, 88
Splitting introducer, for subclavian vein
    catheterization, *15, 16*
SSKI (saturated solution of potassium
    iodide), 18
Stab wound, for gastrostomy, *99*
Stenosis, mitral, 2
Sternal head, *7*
Sternal notch, *7*
  anatomic relations of, *13*
Sternocleidomastoid muscle, common
    head of, *7*
  junction of, *8*
Steroids, chronic preoperative use of, 3
  exogenous use of, hypoadrenalism and,
    4
  perioperative use of, 17
Stoma, for continent urinary reservoir,
    193
  securing of skin for, in rosebud manner,
    194
  site preparation for, in total pelvic ex-
      enteration, *160*
Stomach, anatomic relations of, *96*
  postoperative distention of, prevention
      for, *98*
Strap muscles, *110*
Subclavian vein, anatomic relations of, *7,*
    13
  catheterization of, 6
    for long-dwelling catheter, 20
    incision for vein dilator and intro-
        ducer for, *15*
    J guide wire placement for, *14*
    preparation of operative field for, *12*
    using anterior triangle approach, 6,
        12–15
Subcutaneous external sphincter muscle,
    214
Submucosal tunnel, for distal ureter
    injury repair, *204*
"Sunrise" incision, 108, *118*
Superficial circumflex artery, *37*
Superficial external sphincter muscle, *214*
Superficial transverse perineal muscle, *41*
Superior epigastric artery, *45*
Superior hemorrhoidal vessels, *149*
Superior mesenteric artery, *185, 186*
Superior vesical artery, *55, 166*
Sutures. *See also under specific surgical*
    techniques.
  for closure of Maylard incision, *46*
  for closure of midline incision, *51*
  modified mattress type of, *226*

Tensor fascia lata flap, **240–248**
  borders of, *243*
  closure of, *245–246*
  completed procedure, drainage place-
      ment for, *247*
  drainage placement for, *246, 247*
  indications for, 240, *242*
  overview of, *242*
  postoperative, 248
  potential problem areas of, 240
  preoperative patient preparation for,
      240

Tensor fascia lata flap (Continued)
  radical groin resection for, 243
  rotation of in anterior vulva and groin
    defect, 244
  size of, 240
  suturing of, 248
  transection of, 243
Tensor fascia lata muscle, anatomic
    relations of, 232, 241
Thallium scanning, 5
Theophylline, 3, 17
Thigh, muscular anatomy of, 241
Thigh flap, gluteal, 250
Thoracic artery, anterior, 45
Thromboembolic prophylaxis, 224
Thrombosis, venous, deep, 19–20
Thyroid disease, 4
Thyroid replacement therapy, 17
Thyroid size, physical examination of, 4
Thyrotoxic patient, 17–18
Tilt test, 3
Toldt, line of, 132, 137
Total pelvic exenteration, **140–162**
  anastomosis for, 159–160
  closure of perineal defect with drain-
    age, 155
  completed, with perineal defect, 153
  completion of, in toto, 152
  historical aspects of, 140, 164
  ileal loop isolation for, 156
  lymphadenectomy for, 150
  mobilization of pelvic structures in, 147
  perineal phase of, 153–155
    outline of resection for, 153
  potential problem areas for, 140
  preoperative preparation for, 140
  proximal segment division for, 157, 158
  rosebud stoma for, 162
  stoma for, 161
  stoma location for, 140
  stoma site preparation for, 160
Transverse abdominal incisions,
    advantages of, 44
  disadvantages of, 44
  Maylard incision, 45, 46
    closure of, 46
  operative technique for, 44
Transverse abdominal muscle, 45
Transverse colon, proximal and distal,
    reanastomosis of, 171
Transverse colon conduit, 170–172
Transverse fascia, 109, 110
Transverse incision, for total pelvic
    exenteration, 141
  Maylard-type of, 44, 45, 46, 55
Transverse perineal muscle, superficial,
    154
Transversus abdominis, 114
Transversus fascia, 109, 110
Transversus muscle, anatomic relations
    of, 110, 118, 120
  cutting of, 121
  incision of, 120
Trendelenburg position, for central line
    placement, 12
Tumor markers, 5
Turcot's syndrome, 4t

Ulcerative colitis, 4t
Umbilicus, 118

Ureter(s), anatomic relations of, 59, 68,
    69, 76, 77, 78, 90, 95, 115, 142, 146,
    171, 173
  in rectovaginal space development,
    74
  in reflection of right colon, 132
  in relation to J incision, 112
  in total pelvic exenteration, 147, 149,
    150, 152, 153
  ovarian vessels and, 137
  pulling of, by vessel loop, 122
  uterosacral ligament and, 174
  with ovarian vessels, 128, 130
  with pararectal space, 60
  with pelvic blood vessels, 55
  catheterization of, 148
  dissection of, for radical hysterectomy,
    79
  in radical hysterectomy, 73
  distal, injuries to. See Distal ureter in-
    juries.
  division of, 167
  isolation and cutting of, 148
  left, 191
  retraction of, 95
  right, 191
  separation of, in modified radical hys-
    terectomy, 61–62
  spatulation of, 191, 204
  unroofing of, 63
Ureteral canal, division of, 79
Ureteral catheter, for distal ureter injury
    repair, 206
  for vesicovaginal fistula repair, 199
Ureteral stents, 192, 193, 194
Ureterosacral ligament, deep, 146
Urethra, anatomic relations of, 169
  cutting of, 168
  distal, division of, 167
  from symphysis pubis, 143
Urinalysis, 5
Urinary bladder. See Bladder.
Urinary diversion. See Continent urinary
    reservoir.
Urinary system, monitoring of, for radical
    hysterectomy, 66
Urinary tract reconstruction, 165
Urogenital diaphragm, anatomic relations
    of, 154
  inferior fascia of, 40, 41
Uterine artery, anatomic relations of, 55,
    72, 76, 77
  cut and tied, 101, 165, 166
  ligation of, 175
  medial division of, 93
  transection of, 59
Uterine vein, 55
Uterine vessels, 84, 150
Uterosacral ligaments, 94–95
  anatomic relations of, 60, 61, 141
  clamping of, 166
    in radical hysterectomy, 76
  division of, 103, 166
    for posterior pelvic exenteration, 174
Uterus, anatomic relations of, 67, 73, 74,
    75, 90, 92, 93, 142, 143, 173, 177,
    217
  in relation to rectovaginal fistula, 219
  in total pelvic exenteration, 147, 148,
    149, 150
  dissection of, off rectosigmoid, 103
  removal of, in radical hysterectomy, 82
  with ovarian tumor, 89

Vagina, anatomic relations of, 63, 90, 92,
    93, 94, 169
  in relation to rectovaginal fistula, 219
  in vesicocervical space development,
    75
  angles, ligation of, 102
  closure of, for rectovaginal fistula re-
    pair, 220
  cutting of, for posterior pelvic exentera-
    tion, 177
  defects of, alternate reconstructive
    technique for, 250–262. See also
    specific reconstructive techniques.
  division of, 168
  mucosa of, 217
    closure of, 96
  posterior wall of, cephalad retraction of,
    103
  incision of, 102
  removal of, in radical hysterectomy, 82
  separation of, from ovarian tumor, 95
    from rectum, 210, 219
  wall of, 217, 218
Vaginal cuff, 84
Vaginal hysterectomy, vesicovaginal
    fistulas and, 196
Valvular disease, laboratory evaluation
    of, 5
Valvular heart disease, preoperative
    evaluation of, 2
Vascular pedicle, anatomic relations of,
    235
  for tensor fascia lata flap, 241
  identification of, for gracilis myocuta-
    neous flap, 235
  minor, 233
Vastus lateralis muscle, 232, 241, 244,
    245
Vastus medialis muscle, 241
Vein dilator, for subclavian vein
    catheterization, 15, 16
Vena cava, anatomic relations of, 55, 123,
    124, 129
  in reflection of right colon, 133
  exposure of, 121
  inferior, 112
Venous thrombosis, deep, 19–20
Vertical incision, for total pelvic
    exenteration, 141
Vesical artery, superior, 55, 166
Vesicocervical space, anatomic relations
    of, cross-sectional view of, 75
  development of, 75
Vesicouterine ligament, anatomic
    relations of, 141
  incision of, 62
Vesicouterine space, anatomic relations
    of, 141
  development of, for posterior exentera-
    tion, 173
  dissection of, to vaginal level, 94
Vesicovaginal fistulas, incidence of, 196
  repair of, closed drainage system for,
    202
    for large fistula, 199–200
    incisions for, 203
    indications for, 196
    Latzko partial colpocleisis for, 196–
      199
    Martius bulbocavernosus flap for,
      201–202
    pathophysiologic changes from, 196
    patient position for, 196
    potential problem areas in, 196

Vesicovaginal fistulas *(Continued)*
    ureteral catheters for, *199, 200*
    vaginal approach for, 196
Vessel loop, *122*
Vestibule closure, in rectovaginal fistula repair, *216*
Visceral peritoneum, *142*
Von Willebrand's disease, 5
Vulva defects, alternate reconstructive technique for, *250–262*
Vulvar carcinoma. *See also* Radical vulvectomy.
    early, alternate surgical procedures for, **26–30**

Vulvar carcinoma *(Continued)*
    en-bloc resection of, defect coverage for. *See* Tensor fascia lata flap.
    excision of, 224
    excisional biopsy for, closure of, *30*
        extent of, *26*
        groin incision for, *27*
        indications for, 26
        operative technique for, *28–29*
        pathophysiologic changes from, 26
        potential problem areas in, 26
    groin lymph node dissection for, 26
    incidence of, 34
    local evaluation of, 34

Vulvectomy, radical. *See* Radical vulvectomy.

Xylocaine, *13*

Z-plasty, closure of, *226*
    for defects for vulvar carcinoma excision, 224
    for vulvar lesion excision, *224*
    operative technique for, *224–225*
    physiologic changes from, 224
    postoperative care for, 224
    potential problem areas in, 224